AF432453

Praise for the Work
of Elena Merani, ND, CNHP
and Gregory Hyde, MD, PhD

"What makes the therapeutic experience with Elena and Greg unique and so precious is that it will simultaneously take you into the world of medical science and poetry as a creative act: your body, in fact, will sing a melody, the very personal health story contained in its organs. And the two of them, together, like skilled dancing angels around you, will be able to interpret it by giving word to that sound and restoring its coherence where lost."

--- Dr. Chiara Novaresio, Turin, Italy

"You two are wonderful - just so, so awake, aware, so attuned to the whispers of cosmic intelligence - just brings such beauty to my soul. Every word and nuance is meant to my core...you give light and cosmic love such an incredible boost. You are wind walkers beyond words!!!!"

--- Colleen Brown, Minister/Trauma Release Expert

"I appreciate your intuitive beautiful work ♥ *thank you so much for deeply mirroring my clear true healing to my body so I'm more grounded to support my very subtle vibration insights - such a beautiful expansive dance to be in endless possibility."*

--- Carol Wong, Artist working with Subtle Energy Healing and Creative Arts

Client Testimonials:

I had the pleasure of meeting and being evaluated by Elena and Gregg in October 2019. I apologize for taking so long to write about my very positive experience with them. Based on a strong recommendation from a friend, I drove halfway across the country (750 miles) to see them. When she described what they did, and the tuning forks they used to utilize "sound/vibration" to detect imbalances in the body – I had a "knowing" that I should be there. Their process is definitely "out of the standard medical treatment box" of prescribing drugs (often accompanied with serious side effects greater than the original problem) or surgery (with resulting energy blocking scar tissue) vs getting at the core issue. I have little faith in "Medical box treatments," and so I went.

Walking into the room I could feel their warmth, love of helping humanity, compassion and lightness, and yet it was obvious they both were passionate about their work. I loved the prospect of joining western medical training coupled with sound/vibration/energy medicine in restoring balance to the body without being invasive. I trust the body's natural ability to restore balance when we "listen" to it.

I was amazed and intrigued when they asked me what happened in my life at very specific ages. i.e. 18.75 years old. Every time it was tied to a major event in my life where some traumatic emotional event had occurred. After the third one being "spot-on" – I knew their ability to detect a difference in my body's energy wasn't just a fluke or luck.

As soon as the session began, Elena detected a very deep, deep sadness in and around me which surprised me. I wasn't consciously aware of any sadness. As it turned out, I had taken on deep grief and sadness from my paternal grandmother and also my mother from traumatic events in their lives. Elena cleared that negative/sad energy and I could immediately feel a lightness, a sense of freedom in my chest area. Elena said that I would continue to feel lighter as time went on – and that new opportunities and people would come into my life.

And that has been the case. In fact, I have experienced intuitive guidance and major shifts in my life and have consequently made some key life decisions to move in new and exciting directions (like downsizing and relocating to a new state). I know it was because I was now more open to receive my own inner guidance and be free of this heaviness that Elena said wasn't even MINE! Who knew that we could pick up our ancestor's energy patterns? But it makes sense at some level. And with all the recent changes I've been guided to make that have come about so easily and things falling into place – I'm a believer... and a happy one at that!

They were even able to help me with my sweet Mandy (Bichon Frises dog) who had recently been diagnosed with cancer. They were able to give me a profound message that gave me direction and peace of mind with her eventual passing – which came all too soon and was part of the delay in my writing this review.

In addition, I have had some medical tests done so that Dr. Gregg might help me with my hypothyroidism and not have to take medication the rest of my life. I am looking forward to exploring what may be possible in that area.

I highly recommend these two "trailblazers" who offer so many wonderful gifts. It can be a challenge to describe what they do or what to "expect" because they work on an individual basis – no cookie-cutter treatment sessions here.

Each one is unique as to how your body is vibrating and your energy is flowing.

Treat yourself to the wisdom of your own body that they are able to interpret through the miraculous vibrational tuning forks - along with their uniquely combined intuition and western medical training. Much GRATITUDE to both of you! --- Jacquie Mace

I have traveled the world to see the best doctors to address my serious health challenges. I spent thousands and thousands of dollars in diagnostic testing, prescriptions, and supplements. I also made significant lifestyle changes.

I still didn't feel well.

Continuing to search, I finally found the missing path to my healing--Dr. Greg Hyde and Elena Merani, N.D.!

Their leading-edge methods and incredible knowledge coupled with their Sonic Alignment treatments helped me actually feel better and get better.

I now feel the best I've ever been!

They are truly world-class healing practitioners who made a tremendous impact on my life, more than any other practitioners I've ever seen.

I highly recommend them to anyone who wants to feel their best! --- Julie M., Florida

Healing with Sound

and

The Periodic Table of Emotions

Healing with Sound

and

The Periodic Table of Emotions

Volume I

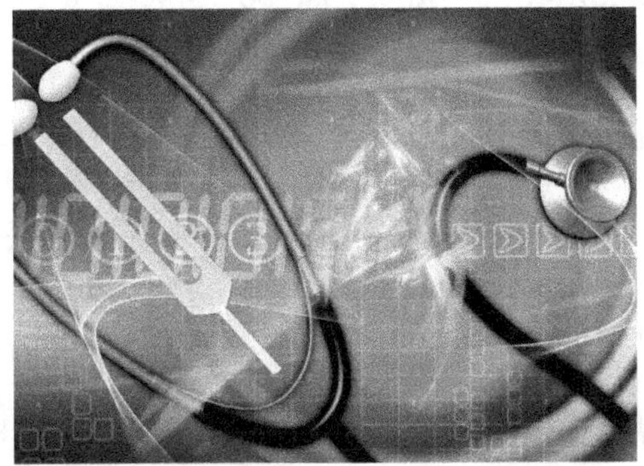

By

Elena Merani, ND, CNHP
Gregory Hyde, MD, PhD

First Electronic Edition: February 2020
First Print Edition: February 2020

Book Design, Formatting and Publishing by
D. D. Scott's
LetLoveGlow Author Services

Indianapolis, Indiana
www.LetLoveGlow.com

I would like to dedicate this book to my husband Greg for helping me trust and believe in myself. Your patience, encouragement and love carried me through my writing journey. I could not have done it without your smile and perfect cappuccino greeting me every morning! Thank you for dancing with me through life and work.

I would like to dedicate this book to my wife Elena for helping me find the courage to change my life and start living my truth. Your unconditional love has healed me in ways I can't describe. Your patience, encouragement, and love has helped my emotionally paralyzed inner child finally start to mature. I still have a way to go, with your help. Thank you for helping me hear my inner song. I love dancing with you through life and work. You are my perfect partner.

Contents

Introduction

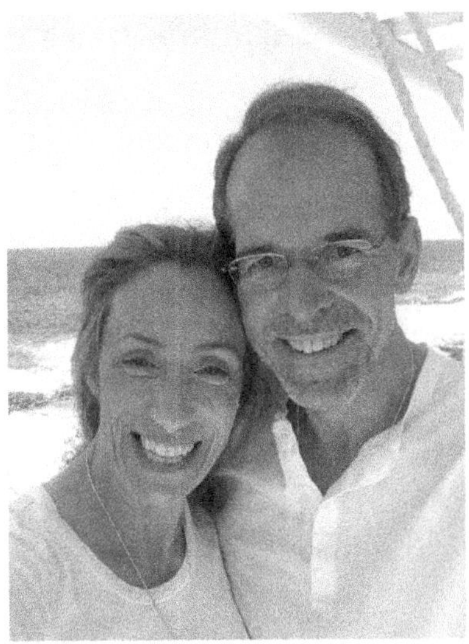

We are humble seekers of truth.

We are open to discovering the beauty and symbolism of the energy vehicle we call the human body.

We believe truth surrounds us in the frequencies that are inherent in every particle of the universe. It is just beyond our consciousness, waiting to be unveiled.

The intention of this book is to open your eyes to information that has been there all along. Over the years, however, our connection to this information and its source has been lost.

We spend an enormous amount of energy and time trying to navigate through what we think we need to achieve to be happy, without realizing that happiness, as we know it, is a reflection of what society has imprinted upon us. In other words, we are told how we are supposed to think, feel and behave in order to be happy; and, as a consequence, we lose ourselves in the process, denying our true nature. Soon we end up living behind a façade of superficial happiness – defined by the society we live in – which throws us out of balance with our authentic self.

Yet, we know something is missing, right?

We believe more and more people are searching for answers about who they are and where they come from.

Ultimately, whether we are aware of this or not, on a deeper level, we all want to know our truth. We are searching for ways to reconnect to our inner self, and we are learning how to replace self-judgment with compassion, appreciation and love. When we find the answers, we have an opportunity to move through life and its challenges with gratitude and grace.

The intention of our work is to help people find their truth by looking at themselves with fresh eyes. We help our clients take a closer look at something that has been there all along, but they haven't been able to see it till now.

It's like using a "magna-finding" glass for the first time and feeling the excitement of seeing the beauty and amazing design of your human body at a whole new level. (Something we were not able to do ourselves until we received the right tools and were pointed in the right direction.)

It is our belief that this information empowers people to recover their original design, and consequently, their health and vitality.

Our hope is that this information will bring a great advantage to a variety of health helpers whose approach is to address the person as a whole, with the intention of integrating mind, body and spirit to help them release dis-ease and discomfort.

It is becoming clear that the chemical, physiological and structural states of the body are deeply connected to, if not regulated by, the energy of our thoughts. In effect, what we think of ourselves (and whether or not our thoughts are in alignment with our natural state) has repercussions/ manifestations in our physical body.

We believe our task here is to follow God's guidance to reveal our work for the benefit of both Natural and Man-Made Medicine. Our hopes are to bridge the gap between Natural, Eastern, and Western medicine. It's about bringing all healing worlds and modalities together versus trying to fight or discredit one or the other.

With Love –

Elena Merani, ND, CNHP
Gregory Hyde, MD PhD
January 2020

Part I

The Hyde-Merani Story
Love at First Tuning Fork

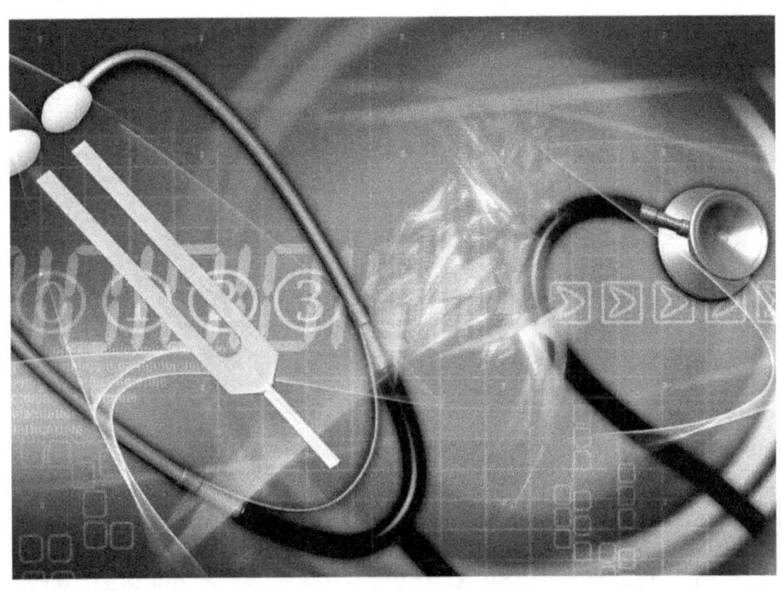

How We Met...Greg's Version

In the fall of 2016, I met Dr. Jerry Tennant at a conference held at Snowbird Resort in Utah. I was impressed with his views on voltage in the body and its role in healing. In the spring of 2017, Dr. Tennant held a Master Course in Dallas. At the time, I was practicing in Eastern Texas, so it wasn't that far for me to travel to attend.

Little did I know that that meeting would forever change my life…

Just after the last break of the meeting, Dr. Tennant announced there would be a special presentation by a visiting Naturopath from Indiana, Elena. She had been working with him in his office for a few weeks. He described how she had used her technique to clear emotional energy from a trauma that no one else had found in his 20+ year quest to heal himself. He had traveled the world trying to regain his own health.

Elena introduced herself as originally being from Milan, Italy. Her English was excellent, and I enjoyed the enthusiastic, animated manner with which she spoke.

She began by asking if anyone in the audience of about sixty doctors and health care providers had ever heard of Biofield Tuning. I raised my hand. It was the only hand raised.

After playing a Native American cedar flute restored my eyesight almost twenty years earlier, I had been actively studying the use of sound in healing. But, that's another story...

Elena glanced at me. I was sitting on the front row, so she could see from my name tag that I was an MD PhD. A slight look of fear came across her face, and she shifted her attention away from me.

She explained what the Human Biofield was and talked about her training with Eileen McKusick, who had written the book, *Tuning the Human Biofield*. I had read Eileen's book and subscribed to her online training videos. Elena had taken her live courses and was a certified practitioner.

She described how she had always loved music and had a gift for languages, which she had studied before coming to the U.S. These traits gave her a unique ability to discern slight changes in the characteristics of sound.

She used a lot of hand and arm gestures as she spoke, typical of the Italian style.

After listening to her for about ten minutes, the thought popped into my head, "She could really use a visual aid."

She had only found out that day that she would have the opportunity to speak at the course. So, I reached down into my computer bag and pulled out a tuning fork I had special ordered. I held it out in front of me, inviting her to use it in her demonstration.

She stared at me in disbelief. And took the tuning fork from my hand.

It served her well for the remainder of her presentation.

She described several clinical cases in which she'd detected hidden dental traumas in teeth, which were causing symptoms and disease in other areas of the body. When the dental problem was addressed, the generalized symptoms resolved. Her clients had nicknamed her "The Tooth Whisperer".

She spoke with great enthusiasm for her quest to try to seek out the root of the imbalance in each of the clients she worked with. I felt a kindred spirit with her in this regard.

At the end of the course, she approached me to return the tuning fork. Since it was one she did not have, I offered it to her. She gratefully accepted it.

I guess you can say that, for us, it was love at first tuning fork!

Elena's Story
The "Why" Question

Growing up I always enjoyed observing the world around me with curious eyes, far more than speaking and engaging in conversations with my friends or family. Those who know me now have difficulty believing I hardly ever spoke as a child, but my older brothers confirm that fact, recalling me saying a maximum of one or two words per week. My husband (Dr. Hyde) still smiles when he hears this, as I am quite the opposite now. I enjoy engaging in conversation and now ask – out loud – a lot of "Why" questions.

My husband asked me one day, "How did you become so wise, Elena?"

"I just ask many 'Why' questions, my dear."

I remember being very shy and scared to venture anywhere outside of a one-meter radius from my mother's skirt. But I loved observing people – how they moved, walked and talked, how every human body was so unique, beautiful and had a secret code hidden inside it.

I don't ever remember thinking that a person had an ugly nose, for example. A nose would just be strong, delicate, thin or long, and I was interested in finding out what that meant.

I realized later that I had a similar outlook regarding nature. My happiest memories as a child were of myself and my family on vacation on The Dolomites. I loved venturing in the open mountain meadows and observing the plants and flowers (their scents, colors and shapes). It felt so peaceful and safe to interact with God's creations. I remember that if I lay flat on the ground, the grass was so tall around me that nobody could see me. It felt good.

But wait…I didn't just observe nature, I was also guided to eat some of the flowers and plants and would think to myself, why am I the only one doing this and why is my mother so upset with me for eating flowers? It seemed so natural to me.

(Note: I learned later in life that there was a reason why, after a meal, I craved a pungent, green-leafed plant with small white flower buds. It was peppermint and its flowers, which are so sweet and delicious when eaten off the ground. My digestive system was calling for a little TLC.)

In the same way, I later learned why I would eat these beautiful, small, purple flowers (bugleweed) as if it was the only food available for the first couple of weeks on vacation. My lungs were in need of detoxing the secondhand smoke I was exposed to in my household during the school year.

But why would I need bugleweed and not any other herb or supplement? Why specifically bugleweed?

For some reason, something about its shape, color, scent and taste resonated with me.

Every plant carries an innate frequency that is a manifestation of a specific emotional and physiological boost our body needs. All creations are out there to support not only our physiological needs but also our emotional ones.

As I was eating bugleweed, feelings of freedom came upon me. My diaphragm seemed to be more open. Bugleweed grows spontaneously in different directions. There is freedom of movement in its pattern, and I really needed to feel free. I needed the freedom of expressing my feelings and developing a sense of self.

This is why it's paramount that, as we develop a protocol for our clients, we take into consideration the emotional components. The physical body is a manifestation of the life experiences and the emotional journeys that our ancestors have gone through.

I remember the first time I took my husband to visit the place I grew up. All of a sudden, I realized, "Wow, why have I never noticed this beautiful building? It seemed so plain and grey before. And what about the view from this balcony?"

After taking a step back and discovering a different angle as a spectator, I saw new opportunities and possibilities.

We can also look at our body the same way…

Observe your body with new eyes. Be excited about what you discover from a different perspective, perhaps from that of your ancestors. Become aware of how beautiful, resilient and powerful it is.

For example, we may think our hips are too big or our nose is not perfect and straight. But, loving our hips or the bump on our nose means to love and integrate all aspects of ourselves. Those hips may have given our ancestors the ability to take on many responsibilities in their lives. That bump on the nose may be a sign of strength and the ability to help others feel safe.

You see? If you understand this information, these traits are each now a GIFT. When we judge and reject or ignore a part of us, we ignore our truth, our essence, and as a result, the body suffers and will try to make us aware of this in any possible way.

Honoring the successes, joys and struggles of our lives is part of our healing journey. However, taking this seat as The Observer of our lives, without judgement, is unfamiliar and uncomfortable. We are creatures of habit, and we like what feels comfortable, even if it's painful.

Most of us are disconnected from our story and the story of our ancestors. Awareness is a very empowering first step, that in many cases, triggers considerable changes in a person's life and consequently changes in their health.

My husband and I give people guidance on how to become aware of the many gifts the body has and the opportunities available to them after recognizing these gifts.

Pain, discomfort and disease are opportunities to discover what has been broken, compartmentalized or judged. This shifts your perspective from feelings of fear to feelings of joy, vitality and empowerment.

Going back to my personal story…

As I grew older, my desire to discover the Whys and How's of the work of our body became stronger. However, Allopathic medicine was not meant to be my path, at first.

I was more interested in understanding what regulates the chemical and physiological reactions in the body. For example, finding answers to questions such as: What is the role of the electromagnetic field in the body? What generates energy to be utilized in one way versus another? What tells an enzyme to shut down or activate? Why are we lacking the building blocks or material that our body needs to function? What regulates what our bodies utilize or reject, incorporate or not absorb?

And…

I believed that thoughts and emotions were part of the driving force that made things happen in the body.

So, I continued to educate myself on human anatomy and physiology and the effects our food and environment have on the body. The scientific studies I pursued in Italy gave me the basis to continue my education through reading and observing the world and the people around me.

Faced with personal and family health challenges that traditional medicine wasn't able to resolve, I decided to start studying Natural Health and became a Naturopath. I studied beyond what the books and lectures had to offer and attended several workshops and seminars on a wide variety of topics.

But still, nobody was able to answer many of my Why questions.

Herbs, supplements and diet alone would bring improvements and a temporary relief in the life of the people I helped, but not a complete resolution of the "imbalance". It seemed also that people would develop a codependency with the supplements they were given by alternative medicine practitioners. They would tell me, "I am well as long as I continue to take my 30 plus supplements a day."

We were still only dealing with the "management" of an imbalance in the body but not with what would help the body restore harmony.

WHY would candida, for example, keep coming back with a vengeance the moment a person would reintroduce even a small amount of sugar in their diet? Or when they stopped taking the supplement that would help keep it under control? What is candida trying to teach us?

Does it have its own meaning and "frequency" just like bugleweed had for me?

Candida, in a small amount, can actually live in harmony within our body. So WHY, for some of us, is it not in harmony anymore? Does every person need a different remedy, depending on their own emotional blueprint? In my opinion, the answer was Yes. That is why the One-Size-Fits-All approach doesn't help everyone.

Guiding others in their journey of self-discovery is the most exciting part of my job!

And when I work with my husband, each individual we meet with is like a gift I can't wait to unwrap.

The joy of a person saying to us:

"Thank you. This is the first time I understand WHY I have been feeling the way I have (WHY I have struggled with candida my entire life),"

or...

"Thank you. This is the first time I have become aware of my inner strength,"

and/or...

"Thank you. I can see my path more clearly than ever before."

Each of these is music to my heart and soul.

Back to what happened after my Aha! Moment that candida is the representation of a frequency that is trying to teach us something…

I realized that we are far more than physical and structural bodies. We are energy and frequency. And if I could figure out the meaning of these frequencies, I would better understand how the body works and what can be done to help restore harmony.

That's the time I started going deeper into the body, studying its electrical and energetic components. All chemical reactions in the body happen thanks to electrical charge. It's what makes the enzymatic function possible.

What switches these enzymes on and off?

Energy.

What creates energy?

Our thoughts and emotions.

And this strongly affects our body chemistry.

Can we identify and integrate, or harmonize, the thoughts and life experiences that affect our ability to establish a healthy relationship with ourselves and our environment (inside and outside)?

How can we help harmonize these frequencies and vibrations of our body in a way that helps us restore our health?

The answer for what we need to help ourselves is, actually, both inside and outside of us, in Nature's creations.

In the summer of 2015, I came across the work of John Beaulieu, a world-renowned speaker, psychologist and composer, also known as an innovator in the field of sound healing. He studied the effects of sound on the nervous system, blood flow and immune response. His work strongly resonated with me and seemed to be the most natural avenue for me as I had been exposed to music as a child, when I started playing classical guitar, and later in life, when I practiced singing and dancing.

Around the same time, I bought a book by Eileen McKusick called *Tuning The Human Biofield*. It was a natural sequel to what I had been learning from John Beaulieu's work. Eileen also had been studying the effects of audible sound on the body since 1996. Her work was eye-opening, and it helped me approach life in a more positive and empowering way.

So, I decided to attend her classes and pursue all the requirements needed to become a Biofield Tuning Practitioner. This laid the foundation of what Dr. Hyde and I developed into Sonic Alignment.

Working and receiving work from other practitioners helped me become aware of the limitations of my own beliefs, of what had been holding me back, of my gifts, my truth and path in life.

I became aware of each person's unique beauty, their undiscovered potential and inner gifts. And I learned that, within each person, every atom, molecule, enzyme, bacteria, and even parasites, have their own beauty and purpose, of which most of us are completely unaware.

In my work in 2016, I was observing how urine pH would change before and after a session. I was curious of the impact on the electrical and energetic body, and stumbled upon the work of a world-renowned ophthalmologist, Dr Jerry Tennant, who, driven by his own difficult health circumstances, was able to uncover the root cause of his condition and find a way to help his body heal through the principle that the body needs *Voltage* to be able to repair, build and heal itself.

To my astonishment, I realized I'd never put two and two together. *This was brilliant!* pH is Voltage, and sound may have a positive effect on the electrical body.

I decided to contact Dr. Tennant, and after visiting his office, I was invited to collaborate in his practice. I worked with sound to facilitate the body's innate ability to relieve stress and reduce resistance to energy flow. This results in empowering people to move forward in various aspects of their life with better ease and balance.

In one of Dr. Tennant's Master Classes, I was asked to give a presentation on the practice of Biofield Tuning. Although I was excited and grateful for the opportunity, I was also very nervous as I was given very little notice, and I found out that most of the attendees were medical doctors or practitioners with years of experience in the medical field. Doing a presentation without slides or any other visual aid was daunting.

I asked if anybody in the audience had ever heard of Biofield Tuning or read about John Beaulieu's work on sound healing, thinking that it would be most unlikely that any of the doctors had heard of either, let alone practiced their techniques. Only one person in the room raised his hand, and he introduced himself as Dr. Greg Hyde, an MD PhD, who had been reading and practicing both techniques since 2015. (Yes, he had started at the same time I did.)

I fell into total panic for a few seconds, imagining the worse scenarios in which this gentleman would start asking all kinds of advanced physics, physiology or acoustical engineering questions.

But to my surprise, he kindly offered me a tuning fork as the visual aid I was missing! *WAIT! How did he know I would be there and needed a tuning fork? My presentation was a last-minute addition to the class.*

At the end of my presentation, he expressed how interesting the twist was that I put into my work and the discoveries that were setting me apart from other sound work practitioners. He shook my hand and gave me one of the tuning forks that he'd had custom made for himself. It was his way of expressing his gratitude for what he had learned from me. The specific frequency numbers of that tuning fork were the three numbers which, in sequence, are my month and birth year.

How did he know that was the tuning fork I had wanted and needed for myself?

Our First Time Working Together

A few months later, Dr. Hyde invited me to assist him in his work, using sound as a supporting aid for one of his longtime clients – Christine.

He had been studying and implementing sound healing techniques from John Beaulieu and Eileen McKusick, as I had been for almost the same amount of time. He also had experience in Native American ways from his own healing journey.

He had been working with Christine for about eight years. During that time, he had gained her trust. She confided in him about some of her early childhood traumas. He felt these were continuing to have an adverse effect on her health, and therefore, requested my assistance.

Something totally unexpected happened...

As we were working together, there was little to no verbal communication between us, except from our interaction with the client; and yet, we were working with sound as if we had been a seasoned, professional tennis doubles pair, practicing and competing together for years.

At the beginning, I worked on an area for a while until there was no progress. Then he took over. When he got stuck, I jumped back in. Ultimately, we began working together in different areas simultaneously which made the session progress even more smoothly.

I wondered, "How can our actions and movements through the use of sound be in such perfect harmony, as if we were dancing a waltz in a ballroom competition?" After all, we barely knew each other.

We found out later that each of us had an amateur dance background. (To this day, we both thoroughly enjoy Latin and Ballroom dancing together. Interestingly, the first time we actually danced together was in front of a former Hungarian National Ballroom Champion. We were considering taking lessons from him in Dallas. "Oh, I see you two have been dancing together a long time," he said. He couldn't believe it when we told him it was actually our first time.)

Back to our session with Christine…

At the end of the session, Christine stood up. She was a little shaky but had a beautiful light on her face and an air of exhausted, but happy relief, similar to a mother giving birth.

"Wow, Dr. Hyde, I think I am having a vision," she exclaimed.

We asked her to share what she was experiencing.

"I see Jesus holding me as a little girl in his arms, telling me I am going to be alright from now on," she said.

After we finished the session and said our goodbyes to Christine, I asked Greg if he had ever witnessed such profound healing before. He said no, he had not. He then asked me the same question. "Never before today," I answered him.

From that time on, more and more people have started seeking our help. It's been an incredible journey of finding out who we really are, both as individuals and as a couple. Together, we have navigated through all kinds of internal and external obstacles which have made our journey more valued and appreciated.

Why I Believe in Sound

Why would an MD PhD with over 20 years' experience in allopathic Western medicine leave his surgical practice to pursue sound healing?

It all started on a Sunday in April 1998…

I woke up with a headache. A really bad headache. This was unusual because I could count the number of headaches I'd had in my life on one hand. I had assignments to do at church, so I decided I could bear the headache long enough to get through the meetings.

While at church, I asked some of the men in my faith to give me a blessing. They laid their hands on my head and told me in their prayer that I would be all right if I did what God expected me to do.

I soon realized that I had also accepted an assignment to do some teaching at another church meeting forty miles away later that afternoon. *Darn.* I really wanted to go home and take something for my headache and go to bed.

Because I wasn't feeling very well, I asked Shirley, my wife at that time, to drive me to the other meeting. There was a tremendous rainstorm, and the windshield wipers quit working on our way there, leaving us blinded by the rain. We pulled to the side of the road, turned off the engine, and said a prayer. When we started the car, the windshield wipers started working again.

I guess I still wasn't going to get out of the meeting. My headache was getting worse. I told Shirley we were going to go get a CAT scan at the ER as soon as the meeting was over.

In the meeting, I was giving my presentation, when I suddenly stopped speaking. After I stood there in silence for about a minute, Shirley felt something was wrong and stood up and touched my shoulder from behind. I immediately fell to the floor and started shaking violently.

I was having a grand mal seizure.

The next thing I remember is a Neurosurgeon standing on the left side of my bed in the ER. He was holding a CAT scan of my brain. He was pointing to a spot on the scan saying, "You have a lesion in your brain right here."

I looked at the scan. I couldn't see it. And I told him so.

"It's right here," he replied, pointing to the scan again.

Again I looked. I couldn't see it. It wasn't like the area was black or missing. I just couldn't see it.

He thought for a moment and then moved to the right side of my bed. Again, he said, "The lesion in your brain is right here."

I looked and saw what appeared to be a tumor in the back of the right side of my brain, the occipital lobe. "Ok, I see it now."

The occipital lobe interprets the visual information that comes from our eyes. The right lobe interprets our left field of vision from both eyes. Because of the lesion in my brain, I had no left field of vision, a medical condition known as a homonymous hemianopsia.

The Neurosurgeon told me I would need to have surgery to remove the lesion in a couple of days, after they stabilized my seizures. He couldn't tell if it was cancer or a parasite or something else. He couldn't tell me if I would ever get my vision back. Then…he walked away.

I was all alone.

I have always believed in the power of faith and prayer. So, I prayed.

I told God that I was willing to accept whatever this was. If my sight never came back, I would not be bitter. I would not fight whatever path this was unfolding. I put my full trust in Him.

The most profound feeling of peace I had ever felt came over me. I knew I would be alright.

I don't remember anything until after the surgery. (Seizures and the medications they give you to stop them don't agree with making memories.)

I remember Shirley and my five children all coming to see me. They all had bald headed skin wigs on so I wouldn't feel like an odd ball.

To my surprise, I didn't have any pain from the large, L-shaped skin incision on the back of my head.

I was told that I didn't have a tumor or cancer, after all. I had an abscess, a pocket of puss in my brain. The organism was streptococcus.

A large catheter was placed into the vein under my collar bone, and I was started on round-the-clock, high dose antibiotics for the next six weeks. They also administered high doses of steroids to try to control the swelling in my brain, in hopes of recovering some of my vision.

After a few days, I was sent home. The left side of my vision was still missing. I started to wonder if I would ever be able to return to work as a surgeon again.

A few days after I returned home, there was a knock at my front door. I answered it. It was my friend, Steve. Steve is a Native American. I was living in Oklahoma, so this was not unusual. Steve had been trained as a Native American Medicine Man. In his hand was a beautiful cedar flute. He held it out to me.

"This is your flute," he said. "It's not like most Native American flutes. You can't buy something like this at a gift shop. This is *your* flute. It is a flute for healing, a Medicine Man's flute. I promise you if you will play it, your vision will come back."

I took the flute. It looked a little like the clarinet I had played for years in band.

I believed Steve. I believed I could play the flute.

It took me several days and several phone calls to Steve to figure out how to get a sound out of the flute. Each time I would call, he would say, "Keep trying. You'll figure it out."

I was used to playing woodwind instruments with a reed. You have to blow fairly hard to get the reed to vibrate. I finally figured out that I had to use very little force to get this new flute to sound. It was more like just breathing. Before long, I could play a scale on the flute and started to make up songs.

We lived on a five-acre lot with lots of blackjack oak trees. I would go outside and sit under one of the trees and play.

The day I first felt I truly played the flute I think I played for about an hour. It was hard to tell. Time seemed to stop. The notes just came to me. I played with my eyes closed.

When I finished, I opened my eyes and looked up into the branches of the tree above me. They were all lined with birds. They were listening to me.

Something miraculous had occurred.

Before I could resume my work as a surgeon, I needed to go get my vision assessed. I wanted to know what residual deficits I had so I could compensate for them and not place my patients at risk. The hospital where I worked also wanted to be sure it was safe for me to resume my privileges there.

I scheduled an appointment with a Neuro-ophthalmologist, a doctor who specializes in the visual portion of the brain. He was located in the Dean McGee Eye Institute at the University of Oklahoma Health Sciences Center in Oklahoma City.

I underwent a thorough examination of my eyes and was placed in a machine to map my visual field. Afterward, I met with the doctor to review my results. He looked at the print-out of my visual field test and said, "Well, that can't be right. Let's run that test again."

I was placed back on the machine again and pressed the button every time I saw the light flash in various parts of my visual field. He picked up the report and compared it to the first one. He had a puzzled look on his face.

I asked if there was a problem.

"Yes and no," he said.

The two reports were identical. And they showed that there were no deficits, at all, in my visual fields. There were no problems with my vision, whatsoever.

The problem was that the doctor couldn't explain why. I should have some deficits, due to the fact that a Neurosurgeon had operated on that area of my brain. I also had an abscess there which should have destroyed some tissue and left residual scarring.

I thanked him for his thorough assessment.

Over the past 20+ years, I have contemplated on the contributions of various factors in the full recovery of my sight. My overwhelming impression is that the sound of the flute played an important role. And I still play it today.

I'm sure the medical treatments I received played a role, although I had a lot of adverse reactions to them. (I had two more hospitalizations within three months that were due to complications of the treatment I received. I firmly believe that if I wasn't a doctor who could challenge some of the medications I was offered, I might not be alive today.)

It was an important learning experience for me. Prior to this illness, it had not occurred to me that I was trying to bring health back to my patients by using poisons. Anything that is labeled "anti" (like *anti*biotic or *anti*-inflammatory) or a blocker (like a stomach acid blocker) is inhibiting a normal function of our body. And there are consequences. I started looking for the consequences in my clients.

I feel it is also important to acknowledge the power of my own faith. I had faith in the men who laid hands on me the morning I awoke with the headache. Faith in the response I felt to the prayer I said in the ER. Faith in Steve's assurance that if I played the flute, my sight would return. Even faith in my Neurosurgeon to allow him to open the back of my head.

I truly believe most of us limit our own healing by our perceptions of what is and isn't possible.

Accepting labels such as *diagnoses* contributes to our limitations. Saying, "I am a (certain) disease" reinforces that disease in our subconscious operating system, making healing more difficult.

And, if the doctor making the diagnosis is wrong, our subconscious can "correct the error" by making that disease occur anyway.

Why?

Because we believe the diagnosis to be true.

I know a man who is the longest living person in Italy with HIV. His response to his doctors who told him he has AIDS has always been the same. "I don't have AIDS."

Bravo!

I have stopped making diagnoses. Instead, I try to reveal temporary problems and imbalances.

Each of us has within ourselves the Gift of Healing.

Most of our gifts are to be used in service of others.

The Gift of Healing, however, is the gift we can only give to ourselves.

As I began learning more about the use of sound in healing, I began to wonder how Steve knew where to put the holes in the flute so that it produced the right tones and frequencies to bring my health back.

It wasn't until about fifteen years after I received the flute, that I learned how it was made. By that point, I had moved away from Oklahoma and was out of contact with Steve.

I was at a medical meeting in Dallas learning about oxidative and regenerative therapies to stimulate healing. I met a man from Santa Fe, New Mexico, and we began talking about our approaches to healing. He was interested in what I was pursuing regarding the use of sound. I invited him up to my room to show him some of my tuning forks. I also had my flute with me.

When we entered my room, he immediately went over to my flute, which was sitting on the dresser. He asked me if he could pick it up and examine it.

"Of course," I said.

He then told me that he collected Native American flutes.

After examining mine for a few minutes, he said, "Wow, this is a unique flute. It's made using The Grandfather Method."

Like I said, I had been wondering how Steve knew where to put the holes. Now, maybe, I would get an answer. I asked him to explain.

"The Grandfather Method uses someone's body proportions to make the flute."

Suddenly, Steve's words came back to me as he gave me the flute. "This is YOUR flute." He had repeated that phrase several times. Now, I had a greater understanding about what he meant.

As we checked, the hole placements were indeed based on my body proportions. For example, the length of the flute from the mouthpiece to the sounding hole at the bottom of the flute was the same distance as the length of my forearm from my middle fingertip to the bottom of my elbow.

This length is called a *personal wavelength*. In ancient times, this unit of measure was called a *cubit*. (Note: You may have seen it mentioned in the Bible.)

If you built your home using your cubit as the standard unit, what would that do to the energy and harmony of your living space? *Just a thought…*

The exact tuning of instruments to specific frequencies is a relatively modern thing. The idea of Hertz is less than 100 years old, first suggested in Germany in the 1920's, but not widely adopted until 1960. (The ability to measure Hertz in sound required the invention of the microphone and modern electronics.)

So much of the current thought on using sound in healing is based on specific frequencies, such as the Solfeggio.

Wouldn't it make more sense to have a sound-based method that is based on the body's geometry and proportions, similar to the way my flute was designed?

Steve had done that for me.

Thank you, Steve. Thank you, wise grandfathers.

Our Aha Moment:
The Periodic Table of Emotions

Working with sound, I began to identify that changes in the tone, timbre and pitch of the tuning fork, accompanied by manifestations both in my mind and body (i.e. a flush or tingle, the vision of a life event, a color or shape) all related to very specific emotions.

Pain, sadness or anger have a very distinct sound that the client can hear as well.

People using sound as a supportive aid to the body's innate ability to heal itself have similar experiences and can relate to what I have described. After some time using sound, we all begin to learn a new language.

As my experience grew and my vocabulary was expanding, I thought it might be interesting to see what certain parts of a plant or flower sounded like. Also, what the sound of minerals, vitamins and even pathogens and toxins sounded like. I thought that they might have their own distinct signature, their own specific sound, but much to my surprise, it turned out that they each share their frequency with very specific emotions.

It became more and more clear that certain minerals are the manifestation of certain emotions. So are vitamins, parasites, toxins and genetic mutations. They all mean something. They are a message that the body is not in balance. It's as if there is a Periodic Table of Emotions as well as The Periodic Table of Elements. And they're designed to work together!

How many times have you tried taking a zinc supplement and you are either still low in zinc, or your levels drop the moment you try to stop taking it?

Why does this happen?

When you understand the meaning of zinc, you will realize why. Even if your body has absorbed it, it hasn't been able to keep up with the demand for it. You will also understand why there was an assimilation issue in the first place.

Some people use great amounts of courage in their daily life. Others work in jobs that require a lot of patience, for example. A great need for courage or patience explain why they may be deficient, or in need of the mineral or nutrient that relates to these emotions. They may even need more of it than normal.

On the other hand, some people are deficient in a certain mineral because they have never integrated the emotion connected to that mineral. It has been "broken" or compartmentalized since the time of a personal or ancestral trauma.

Genetic mutations also carry their own emotional signature and create imbalances and deficiencies in the body.

The point is to become aware of each mineral's meaning and of the lessons you are here to learn from it. Once the lesson is learned, the body can change.

The beauty of this discovery is realizing that it is ok sometimes to be low in zinc. You may be using a lot of the emotion related to zinc. Don't judge it or be impatient to change it right away. Just observe it at first and be grateful for what your body has been through. Then you can reintroduce that frequency with the knowledge of what it means and what it does for you. At some point in the past, that knowledge was either lost or broken.

The next question is how do we balance or harmonize these minerals?

The solution depends on each person's emotional composition. And that is different for each one of us.

Think about my initial example with bugleweed. There are many remedies used for cadmium detoxification (from the secondhand smoke I'd been exposed to). But only one was the right one for me, because it harmonized an emotion related to a trauma that had not been processed well when I was a child.

Even bacteria and viruses, which are part of us, don't necessarily need to be destroyed or eliminated. Again, we need to understand why they are "having their way with us" and what they are trying to tell us. Otherwise, even though treated with medication, they will continue to come back (like strep infections, for example).

The immune system needs to re-establish a healthy relationship with the microbe at issue by acknowledging that we have heard the message that it's trying to send us.

If we fail to acknowledge the message, we lose connection with our body and its identity. This results in an abnormal, hypersensitivity reaction to the microbes, which is the basis of auto-immunity. (We'll discuss this more in another chapter.)

Through the use of different sound modalities and the Sonic Alignment technique, we have learned to identify the relationships that need to be repaired and re-established. By bringing the emotional context to our clients' awareness, they are able to acknowledge their body's condition and set in motion the changes that will result in a return to more balanced function. We can then restore the body's immunologic relationship with its microbes and lessen auto-immune inflammatory reactions, using an advanced form of immunotherapy.

Part II

The Periodic Table of Emotions
(Minerals, Vitamins, Microbes, and Toxins)

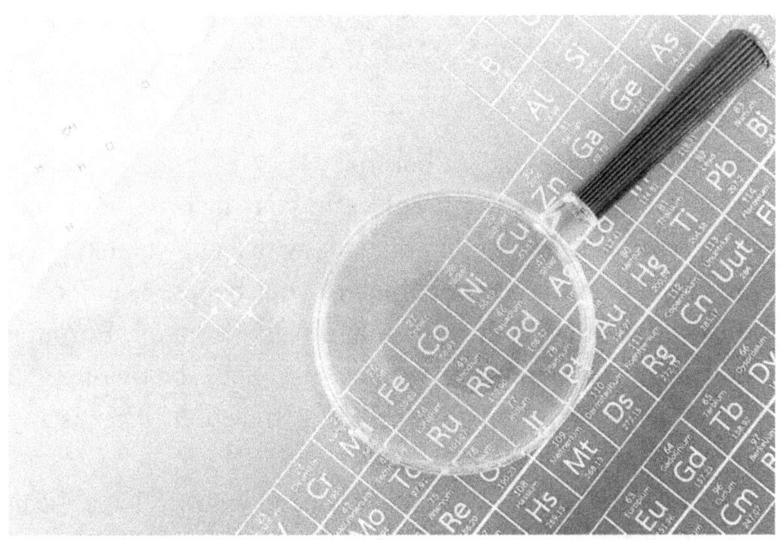

BORON – Belonging
(Security of Territory)

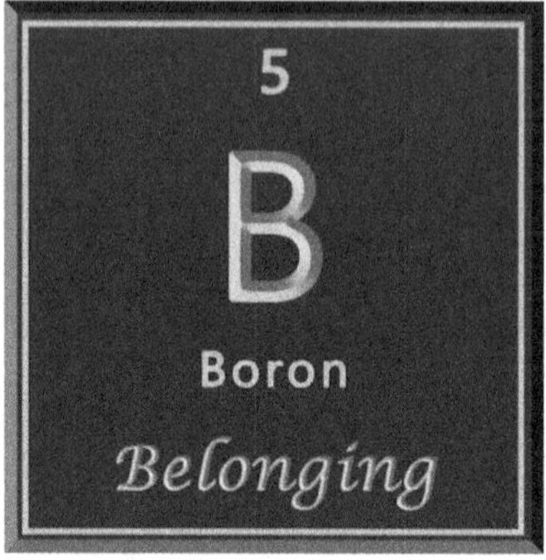

What is the "feeling" of boron?

It's like sitting by the fireplace in your favorite room and feeling your body sink into your sofa with a cozy blanket. It's cold outside, and you feel chilled to your bones. The door to the room is closed with a "Do not disturb" sign on. Boron is reminiscent of warmth, grounding and belonging. It proclaims, "Everyone, I am taking a time out. This is my territory. Please do not trespass!"

In our work on teeth, my husband and I, have been particularly attentive to all the factors that contribute to a healthy mouth. This is a sensitive subject for me, since I lost most of my molars and always wondered what could have been the possible contributing factors, both physical and emotional. Using sound to listen to teeth has been a mission of mine for the last five years, and it earned me the nick name, "The Tooth Whisperer".

First, I would like to make it clear that what I am going to present here is not the only factor that determines the health of your teeth, but it is certainly a contributing one.

My diet has always been balanced and based on whole, natural food. I have always flossed and brushed my teeth diligently. On the other hand, I have come across people in their 50s and 60s, who use, at most, just a toothpick to clean their teeth and certainly don't hold back on sweets, and they don't have a single cavity. Something just didn't add up.

Last summer, I started observing something very interesting while gathering data on clients who had experienced several cavities at a young age and others who lost many teeth, if not almost all their teeth, as young as in their late 30s and 40s. They were all born or lived in Europe, and they all manifested a significant decrease in boron levels in the body at a VERY specific time in their life. For some of them, that time corresponded with the end of 1982, but for the majority, it was with the end of 1986, with levels continuing to drop rapidly in 1987.

My husband and I looked at each other in astonishment. *Pazzesco*! (*Crazy!*)

Those years correspond to the two Chernobyl meltdowns. The first accident in 1982 was ignored for years, but the second one was more devastating and difficult to cover up. You can find videos which show how the cloud of radiation stretched as far as France to the West and England to the North, with most of the damage in the Eastern European countries.

Boron is used in nuclear reactors to absorb and neutralize radiation. Our bodies also need boron, however, in its effort to release radioactivity contamination and the effects of radiation. Another very important function of boron is to facilitate the metabolism and absorption of calcium, magnesium and phosphorous. Low boron levels in the body have a significant impact on bone density and tooth mineral composition.

Interestingly, we notice a similar effect of boron deficiency in the food we eat.

Have you ever noticed the brown, soft tissue near the core of an apple when you slice it? It looks firm and intact on the outside, it's even crispy when you take the first bite, but it is soft and brown near the core. The core of the apple dries out and forms larger cavities. And the pulp is not as dense. That's boron deficiency! Teeth also may seem healthy on the outside but the bone around the root may be soft and not as dense as it should be, and this has an impact on tooth mineralization.

Radiation exposure, smoking and other environmental toxins play a considerable role in the health of our teeth, but I believe that emotional trauma has the biggest impact of all.

Lack of Boron carries its own emotional signature. It means lack of boundaries and the loss of a territory in which we feel safe.

Many people in Eastern Europe have suffered persecution under a dictatorial regime and experienced a sense of rejection. Many felt and still feel like they don't belong to their native land, that they have to leave their country or home and travel like gypsies. They have been on a quest to find their home/roots and learn to establish boundaries in their lives.

Before you jump to the conclusion to run to your local health food store and buy a boron supplement, you need to be aware that not every source of boron is created equal. Just taking a vitamin high in boron isn't always the solution. The food with the highest concentration of boron is root vegetables. But here's the tricky part…which root vegetable is best for YOU? The answer depends on your emotional profile.

This is a big part of our work with each client privately…exploring/discovering their emotional profile so we can then propose which type of boron-infused substance is the best for them as an individual. The shape, color, taste and even location where the food or herb is grown can make a huge difference on the bio-availability and utilization of boron for each person.

A capsule is usually not the best answer.

CALCIUM – Protection

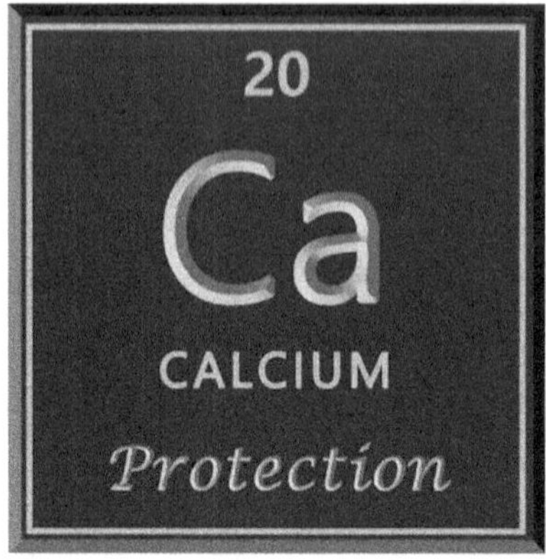

Did you ever enjoy climbing trees or playing in a tree house? For some of us, it was the secret escape where we could be ourselves, where we felt in control and free to let go of our creativity.

Calcium feels like a solid tree house built in an oak tree. A place where we are free to be ourselves and are protected from predators. (Interestingly, oak bark and stems are very high in calcium.)

Calcium also gives the feeling of being inside a shell.

And think about it…what are shells made of?

Calcium.

A client once described visualizing herself shrinking to the point of being able to dive into a spiral-shape shell, where she felt safe, protected and "FREE OF JUDGMENT". She could be sheltered, while still allowing movement in her life, just like shells move with the tide and rhythm of the ocean.

In our work, we found that one of the physical manifestations of growing up in a highly judgmental environment and having to comply with high expectations and strict rules can disrupt our relationship with calcium.

Calcium may not be fully absorbed and utilized. It can even fall out of solution and create calcifications in the body. The person may manifest muscle tightness and rigidity of movement, as well as resistance to change, attachment to firm beliefs, control of themselves and others, and a fear of judgment.

The result is living mostly in fight or flight or protection mode, where there is little to no movement in our lives, and we feel like our real self has no avenue of manifestation, or worse, we don't even know who our true self is.

How do we protect ourselves from our own judgment and our own fears?

Our body responds in many ways, depending on what it is that we are judging or are fearful of.

The interesting part of our work is that it has allowed us to discover that, just like minerals, different types of bacteria, viruses and toxins also correspond to different emotions, which we have mapped and are excited to share.

Most of the time, our immune system keeps the bacteria "under control", and they live in a symbiotic relationship with our body, but…when we judge the emotions related to a specific bacteria, our body will "release" calcium from our bones to build a protective wall around it. It protects us from our own judgment!

When we listen to areas of calcification in the body (gallstones, kidney stones, arthritis, etc.), we find undigested emotions and traumas which share the same frequency of a toxin or bacteria that the body "walled off" with the intention to protect itself.

We believe that being aware of who we really are and uncovering our truth WITHOUT JUDGMENT is a very important step that allows our body to manifest harmony and bring healing.

What helps balance Calcium in our body?

As with Boron, simply taking a supplementation can often make the problem worse. Again, it depends on what the calcium is trying to protect you from.

One mineral is particularly important to offset the often over-protective, over-controlling quality of calcium. And that is Magnesium.

We'll get the "feel" for Magnesium next…

MAGNESIUM – Spontaneity

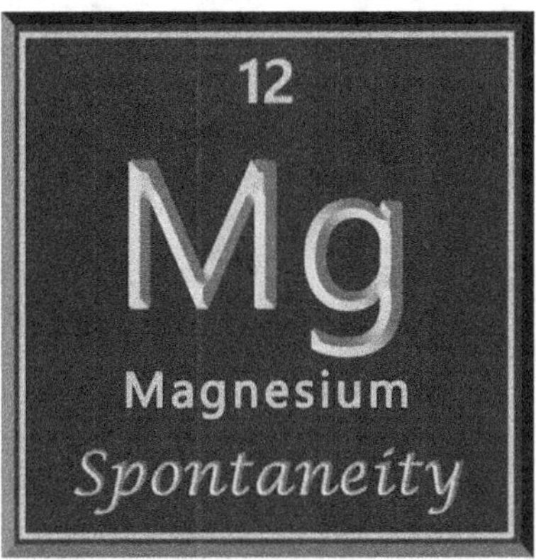

Imagine yourself relaxing by the beach, soaking up the sun and listening to *"Groovin on a Sunday Afternoon"* by The Rascals. You are not worried about what time it is or what you will do next, instead you are wondering if you should take a dip in the water, sunbathe or sit in the shade and read a book. You don't have to be in control, you are just relaxed and follow the rhythm of the sun.

Magnesium is the quintessential "chill" mineral and allows us to live in the moment.

Have you ever observed how the leaves of a plant move spontaneously through the day, positioning themselves to be optimally exposed to the sun?

Chlorophyll, the green substance in leaves, is used to utilize and convert energy from the sun into sugars (carbohydrates) by combining carbon dioxide and water.

Chlorophyll requires magnesium to function, and it represents spontaneous movement through the day, and similarly, that same kind of spontaneous movement through our lives.

It is interesting that our human bodies require magnesium to reverse this process – the process of converting sugar back to energy forms that our cells can use. We release carbon dioxide and water in the process, completing the beautiful cycle.

What happens when magnesium has not been integrated or processed correctly by our body?

We have observed that people are more likely to bottle up or repress their emotions, but then, all of a sudden, they have an unpredictable, emotional outburst of anger and aggression. They may also experience considerable anxiety and fear, which comes in many forms, such as the fear of pain, fear of loss and separation of a loved one (which ultimately prevents them from fully enjoying each moment with them).

On a physical level, we have seen that organ calcification, high blood pressure, stiff muscles, cramps, headaches, nervous system disorders and even depression can be manifestations of low magnesium.

We have observed that people suffering from the above conditions often experience repressed emotions, unexplained or unfounded fears, and lack of spontaneity in their lives. They feel like they don't have control of their lives.

Part of these people's operating systems, at some point in their lives (or the lives of their ancestors), went off track.

We recently had a client with low magnesium who lost her mother when she was two years old. Her mother was in her 30's when she died of polio, a viral illness which results in muscle stiffness and paralysis.

Shortly before the onset of the polio virus, her mother had learned that her husband, our client's father, had developed multiple sclerosis and would likely die.

When we listened to our client's mother at the time she had polio, there was the sound of an extreme deficiency in magnesium.

We were curious if there was any known relationship between low magnesium levels and susceptibility to polio. We found a 1948 publication by a physician who had successfully stopped the polio disease and restored movement to paralyzed limbs by administering magnesium salt (MgCl) to a number of patients soon after the onset of symptoms.

The despair, lack of control, and sadness that this mother suffered at the time she found out her husband would die had triggered a rapid loss of magnesium which made the body more susceptible to disease.

Sound helps us identify why and when relationships have gone off track. It helps us become aware of these variables. And then, nature again can be a way to bring balance to the bodies of those with these issues.

So…should these people start eating large quantities of spinach and field greens (which are high in magnesium)? Pop magnesium capsules in their mouths? Or are poppy seeds the answer (also high in magnesium)?

The truth is within each of us.

We just help you uncover what that truth is for YOU.

God helps us find YOUR answer.

Vitamin B1 & the Right Foot

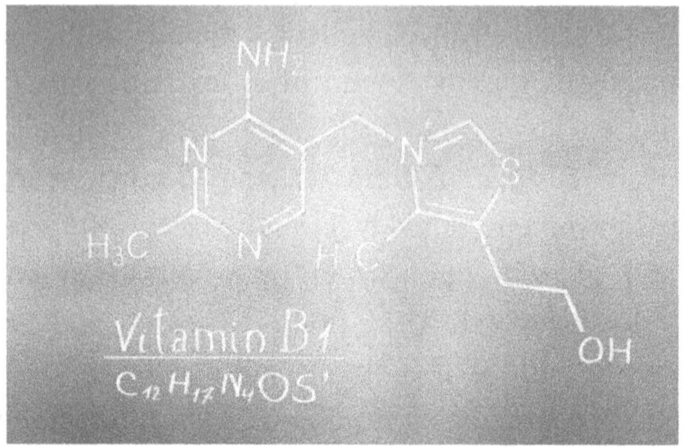

Elena was listening to me one day with her tuning fork. She does that with me, a lot, usually at times I am not aware she's doing so. She reminds me frequently that she fell in love with my sound before she fell in love with me.

On this particular occasion, she found something she had never heard before in me. As she evaluated my nutrient levels, she found the sound related to my Vitamin B1 level was very low.

I eat very well and usually take a multivitamin with a good dose of vitamin B1, so I was very surprised by her finding. However, I knew from past experience that when she has found low B vitamin levels in our clients, it was true.

When she listened to my electric body, I had a lot of heaviness in my right foot. It was making the same tone as my low B1 level on her tuning fork. When we find a particular frequency in one area of the body, we will then scan the rest of the body to see if we can detect the same frequency somewhere else. In this way, we can determine if the two findings are related or not.

She recalled that she had found low Vitamin B1 levels in other clients who also had energetic heaviness on their right foot. They also had many other findings that masked the relationship. Consequently, she had not recognized that the two findings were related. Because these were new findings that had not existed in me before, she was able to recognize the association.

She asked me if I had been having any problems with my right foot starting about ten days ago. Upon reflection, I remembered that there had been intermittent, brief twinges of pain, but only when I stressed my foot by running. And yes…this had first appeared about ten days prior.

It wasn't causing me to limp. I just was aware that something in the center of my foot had changed.

Then Elena asked me what vitamin B1 does in the body. I had studied biochemistry as an undergrad, so I knew what thiamine, the chemical name for B1, does. Thiamine, along with alpha-lipoic acid, are cofactors in the FIRST STEP of the Krebs cycle. The Krebs cycle is the name of the sequential chemical reactions that take place in the conversion of glucose into CO_2 and water as ATP is produced. ATP is the energetic currency that empowers us to move.

Symbolically, the right foot is all about taking a FIRST STEP, setting out on a new project, or starting something fresh and new. When we acknowledged this "first step" symbolism, we both got angel bumps. I was working to secure new medical licenses, generating content for our website and starting to write this book. Lots of first steps going on simultaneously. Maybe too many for the small amount of B1 I was consuming.

Elena's intuition told her there was a food that would help me. She felt like the energy needed to come from a food that was round. That is the geometry of an egg or seed. She researched which foods are highest in vitamin B1/thiamine. She found lentils and black-eyed peas high on the list. And both are round.

We had another aha moment. Followed by more angel bumps.

Elena grew up in Europe. They have a tradition there that, every New Year's Eve, you have lentils with your meal. I had lived in the Southern US for nearly 25 years. There, you have black-eyed peas on New Year's Day. Both traditions are for the fresh start of the New Year, another FIRST STEP moment.

I'm still eating lentils...

Part III

Roadblocks to Your Health

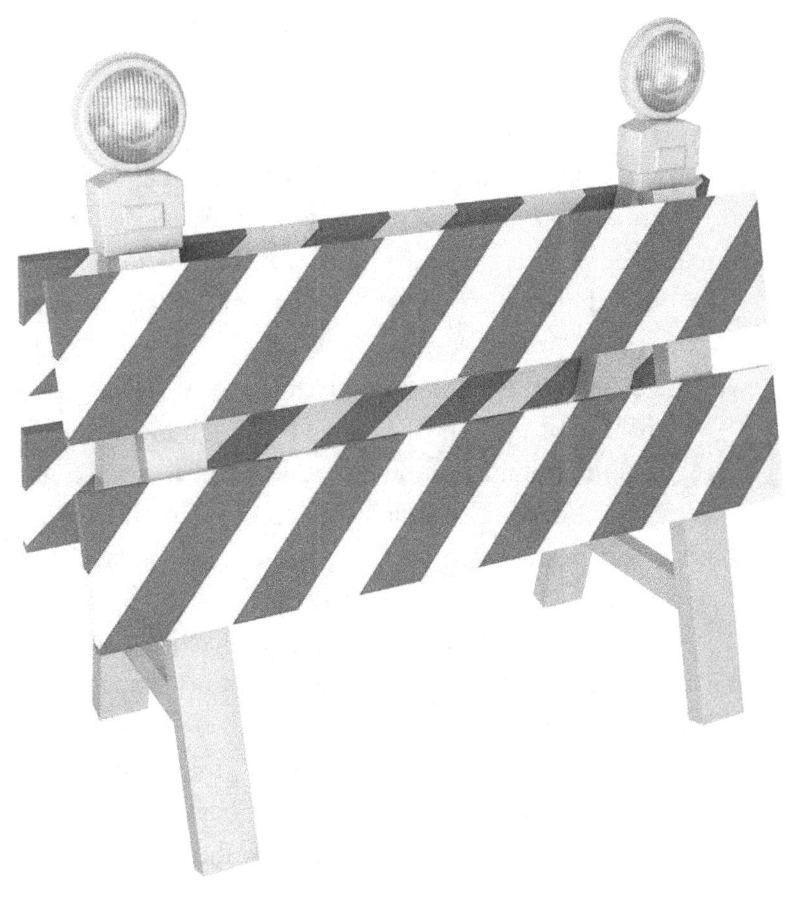

Emotional Scars

Ever notice how some scars heal really well and others never quite look like they finished healing?

There could be emotions stuck in the scar.

Here's how I know...from my personal experience…

An Adverse Childhood Event

When I was three years old, I was asleep in the back of my parent's Nash Rambler when they were struck head on by an oncoming car. It was Memorial Day Weekend, and we were on our way to visit my grandparents in Idaho.

In 1962, there were no seat belts or children's car seats.

I became a projectile inside the car, flying over the front seat and striking the metal dashboard with my face.

My father put the top of his head through the windshield, nearly scalping him. My mother cut her right eye and legs.

We were taken to a small Emergency Room where the doctors addressed my parents' injuries first as they were more severe.

I had lacerations across my right forehead at the hairline and down the full length of the left side of my nose, from the bridge to my cheek.

The doctors had been very busy that night in the Emergency Room, with lots of lacerations, including ours. When it came time to repair my wounds, they found they had no more local anesthetic.

So, they wrapped me up in a papoose, a pediatric immobilization device, and had my mother hold me down while they sewed up my face. *It was all they could do. I know that.*

I remember the sterile drape coming over my face before they started sewing.

Ever since then, I have not liked anything close to my face, especially something resembling a cloth or drape. For example, I can never pull the covers up over my head for very long. If I try, waves of anxiety overcome me. When I started SCUBA diving, wearing the face mask sometimes caused the same response.

As a surgeon, I have to wear a surgical mask. Every time I put one on, I close my eyes and imagine a calm happy place so I can stand to wear it. Usually by the end of the procedure, though, my nervous system has started to revolt and release adrenaline. And when you're a surgeon, shaking hands are a problem.

Repressed Memories

I didn't realize that my aversion to things near my face was related to my childhood accident until 1998. I had forgotten most of the details of the accident.

My reactions to cloth or drape-like materials near my face were a defense mechanism from my subconscious. My subconscious was telling me, "It wasn't much fun the first time. Why would you ever want to think about it again?"

But, evidently, in 1998, my subconscious finally felt like I was ready to start dealing with some of the truth.

That was the year I had a brain abscess that took away half my vision. As I was recovering, I started dreaming about my childhood accident.

I wrote down what I remembered about being sewn up without anesthesia and shared it with my mother. Her response was, "You were so young then. We hoped you wouldn't remember."

How could I not remember?!

Every day since the accident, when I looked in the mirror, I would see the scars on my face from the accident. The scar on my forehead was always raised above the surrounding skin, and it was reddish colored. The one down the left side of my nose was flat, but dark brown, hyperpigmented.

I thought the dark coloration was due to the scar getting too much sun the summer after the injury. I actually used the scar as a visual aid for my plastic surgery patients, warning them to wear their sunscreen after surgery or they would look like me.

Knowing my aversion to wearing a surgical mask was related to the accident allowed me to release some of the emotional energy. I forgave the doctors in the ER and my mother.

My anxiety about having things close to my face improved, but didn't completely resolve. I had released the energy from my mind, but not the scar.

It wasn't until 2014 that I learned scars hold emotional energies and how to release them.

Emotional Scar Release

I was doing some internet training on a new energy device I had just purchased – the Ondamed. The presenter, who was from Germany, mentioned the name of a German physician who now practices in the United States, Dr. Dietrich Klinghardt, MD PhD.

I had never heard his name before. But it shot through me and made such a strong impression that I stopped the recording and immediately did an internet search on him. I found his website and read his views on healing. I also watched some of the video links on the site.

I was surprised to find that we shared many of the same views and approaches to health and healing. I knew I had to meet him and learn more from him.

The next morning, I called his organization to see when his next training course might be. The woman who answered the phone told me he had a five-day retreat on Whidbey Island in Washington State in two weeks, but it had been sold out for months. However, just that morning she had been notified of a cancellation so there was one seat left. I took it.

I had goose bumps as I hung up the phone.

The location of the conference was right across the bay from the city where I had grown up, Everett, Washington. I was going home.

Dr. Klinghardt uses his annual retreat to teach his healing techniques by allowing the participants to become patients. I was introduced to many new aspects of energy healing and the role that emotions play in causing disruption to our health. It was a turning point in my health and my approach to healing.

One of the methods he taught us is a German technique known as Neural Therapy. It is currently widely used in German-speaking countries as part of their everyday care of patients. However, it is almost unheard of here in the U.S.

Scars frequently cross the energy meridians of the body. Surgical training does not teach how to avoid injury to this part of our physiology nor how to restore the lost function.

Neural therapy uses a short-acting, local anesthetic – procaine – to restore energy flow across scars and traumatized areas of the body. It does so by resetting the nervous system's response to the injury.

Some effects can be immediate. I have seen it restore full range of motion to joints that were frozen after surgery, sometimes for years, within minutes after the treatment.

At the Klinghardt course, I felt strongly that I needed to have the scars from my childhood car accident treated.

As the procaine was introduced superficially into the brown scar on my nose, I was suddenly transported back to that ER room in 1962. Every sensation I had at that time was present, including all the emotions: the fear, the pain, the anger, the struggling to escape, the surrender.

I was three years old again.

I spoke to the staff who were treating me as that scared, traumatized child. I vented emotional energies that had been suppressed for over 50 years. I was supported and guided until it felt like everything had cleared.

I felt a calmness inside me I had been missing.

The next morning, I looked at myself in the mirror. To my amazement, the scar down the side of my nose was no longer dark brown. It had almost completely disappeared.

I feel the color was an indication of the dark emotions being held there.

When the dark emotions left, so did the dark color.

So, Now What Do I Do?

When I returned from my retreat with Dr. Klinghardt, I was a very different person on a very different path. I am grateful to him and those I met through his courses who have encouraged my change.

My experience with my own scars left me concerned about the effect I was having on my patients. After all, I am a surgeon – one who creates physical scars on a weekly basis.

Surgery Unplugged: The Acoustic Version

I had already learned during my brain abscess illness in 1998 that emotions like anger and resentment could cause pain when trapped in a wound. The pain could be reduced or eliminated by forgiveness. (I plan to share the full story at a future time.)

For the next 20 years of my career, I tried to always remember to ask my patient's forgiveness for any pain I might cause them, usually before I caused it.

I would say, "If I hurt you, will you still be my friend?"

"Sure, Dr. Hyde" was their usual answer.

The children I operated on would usually give me a hug.

During the operation, I would do everything I knew to lessen the pain response and minimize trauma to the area of surgery.

I worked hard to control my emotions and have a cooperative, positive, supportive environment in my operating room.

During the surgery, after the patient was asleep, I would silently ask their body's permission to operate. When I felt I had it, I would proceed.

(Note: Surgery needs to be conducted in a sacred space. Anesthesia and sedation make the body more vulnerable to all the energies in the environment. I'll share more about this shortly...)

I would try to hold love, gratitude, and forgiveness in my heart as I worked. To the extent that I was successful, my patients reported little or no pain after surgery.

The ultimate proof I was making a difference came when I performed a tonsillectomy on my 19-year-old son, Leighten. He had a rough Freshman year of college, due in part to frequent tonsillitis. His tonsils were very enlarged and filled with pockets of infection.

A tonsillectomy when you are a child can be very traumatic and painful. It certainly was for me at age 4. A tonsillectomy when you are an adult can be one of the most painful experiences you can imagine.

During his surgery, I was distracted at the beginning. It is not easy operating on your own child. But I felt I could do it less painfully than any other doctor I knew.

I had already removed his right tonsil when I realized I had not connected with his body and was not holding the right attitude as I operated.

I stopped, connected, and asked forgiveness through my heart before I removed his left tonsil.

He stayed at home after the surgery, so I was able to check on him every day. I finally got the courage to ask how his pain was on the second day.

He replied, "Not that bad, Dad. But why does it only hurt on the right side?"

I explained to him why and asked his forgiveness.

He gave me a big hug.

Adding a Fork to My Knife, A Tuning Fork

Over the past five years, I have treated hundreds of clients with Neural Therapy. For the past three years, it has been combined with Sonic Alignment with Elena's help. The combination of sound from the tuning fork and procaine into the scar appears to have more profound and lasting results.

When I first treated a scar on Elena, she released grief from the loss of her mother at age 38. She hadn't been able to process any emotions at her funeral and had repressed them for many years.

Her sobbing was so loud I was afraid people in the building would think I was harming her. It continued for over ten minutes. She still tells me it was the most profound emotional release she has ever had.

That experience early in our relationship made her see me and my medicine in a much different way.

Whose Emotion Is This?

The emotions that are carried in the body are not always our own. We frequently find the emotional patterns of the ancestors of our clients stuck in the areas we are helping.

We believe the DNA transfers these energy patterns to the water of the body. (More on this in our second book.)

Pets pick up the emotional energies of their owners. They tend to lie on or next to the areas of the body that need the most help. (Note: We frequently "tune up" the family pets to lessen their load.)

Children do the same thing for their parents, especially before adolescence. Emotions experienced by the mother during pregnancy are strongly transferred to the developing fetus. After all, they are one being during gestation.

Did Your Surgeon Leave Something Behind?

We have found the emotions of the surgeon present in scars on several occasions.

Elena referred a client to me (we'll call him DT) after she found a lot of sadness in a scar on his wrist where carpal tunnel surgery had been done. DT had not been having any major emotional events in his life at the time of his surgery.

Whenever he gripped something, he had pain radiating from the scar to his elbow. The pain started after the surgery. His surgeon couldn't explain why.

Elena listened to his wrist, focusing on the day of the surgery and sensed a change at about 9 a.m. DT said that was when the surgeon made the incision.

She then noticed tremendous sadness pervading the room at that time. She asked DT if he knew anything about the surgeon's personal life. And…he did.

The surgeon had shared with him, in the pre-op area, that his wife was dying of cancer.

Elena and I helped DT clear the sadness from the scar using Sonic Alignment and Neural Therapy.

The pain in his arm resolved and his grip strength returned.

The Weakest Link

We have found that emotional energies seek out the weakest areas of the body. Frequently, these areas are external scars. But they can also be internal scars in joints, ligaments, muscles, bones, or organs that have been damaged.

The emotional energies further interfere with the flow of energy and information in the area where they coalesce. In essence, they form an energy cyst which acts as a blockade to normal energy flow and function.

Pain is a message from our body that energy is not flowing, and function is being affected.

As we were developing our skills with Sonic Alignment, we would frequently have experiences where the pain in an area of the body would resolve during our session.

We would be happy. Our client would be happy.

Then the pain would re-appear in a different area, the next weakest one in their body. *Nuts!*

When we first started working together, we would chase the pain around the body, like trying to catch a chicken. Fortunately, we have learned more effective ways to get the energies to exit the body, rather than just relocate.

Energy cannot be destroyed. It can only be moved or transformed.

Using Sonic Alignment, along with other techniques such as Neural Therapy, we have empowered our clients to restore areas of their health that they thought had been lost and had thus given up all hope of healing.

Immune System

Our Immune System is the receiver of the thoughts and opinions we have of ourselves. And a lot of this is imprinted through our DNA and molded by our environment as a child.

But also…our Immune System is about how we honor and respect ourselves.

For example:

- The thymus gland responds to our answer to the question 'Am I truly being me?'.
- The spleen is all about how we love and nourish ourselves and whether we keep ourselves in high value (in other words…our self-esteem). Elena calls it "self-espleen".
- The appendix is governed by how well we accept our so-called "mistakes," the choices we make or fail to make, and imperfections in our physical appearance. Guilt and shame resonate here.

We have been created to honor our gifts. The life we were given, and its purpose, is the first one of these gifts. Our wishes and desires are additional gifts, along with our ability or choice to accept our struggles and learn from our mistakes. We need to develop unconditional love for every aspect of ourselves, including our appearance.

When we negatively judge our physical, emotional and spiritual self, our Immune System greatly suffers. It doesn't know who is the authentic you. It doesn't know the difference between who you are and who society wants you to be. What a perfect storm for autoimmune diseases!

The physical manifestation of our gifts and our authentic self are our good bacteria, red blood cells, immune system, minerals and vitamins.

But there are also physical manifestations of our "mistakes" and our process of learning lessons and the "ugly" part of us, the parts we are ashamed of.

You know what that is?

It's bacteria, viruses and parasites, which are also there to teach us a lesson. And yet, we believe we need to "eliminate" these lessons.

Here's how it works…

Are we speaking for ourselves? Are we speaking our true, authentic voice? Do we feel like we are being heard? Are we ignoring our inner voice?

If we are not, the very bacteria (Streptococcus) that normally lives undisturbed in our throat, as part of our normal flora, will wake up and decide to build a fire in our body (as Dr Hyde describes it) to get our attention. It literally will build a fire in our throat and make our throat miserable for a few days, with the hope that we will listen and learn the lesson.

Strep is not the enemy. It's the part of us that acts much like a conscience, giving us notice that we are moving out of integrity with ourselves. If we don't listen to our body, eventually that fire will turn into a more serious condition.

Here's another example…

Am I standing my ground? Do I have a foundation of truth for my body? Do I respect myself?

If the answers to these questions are 'no', Helicobacter pylori (H. pylori) bacteria uses the frequency of its shape to make us aware that we need to ground ourselves, digging our roots deeper into our authentic self.

H. pylori is a corkscrew-shaped bacteria that "screws" into our tissues and has roots on one end. It is estimated to infect over half the world's population.

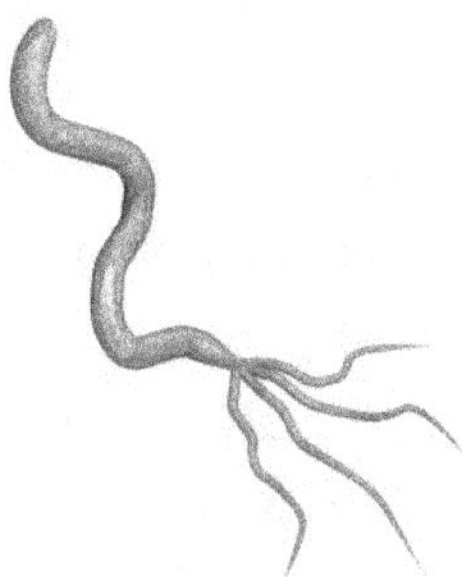

Its corkscrew shape allows it to dig and root into us when we're out of resonance with our personal truth, causing us such dis-ease as stomach ulcers and cancer.

Once we become aware of this lesson, the H. Pylori will say, "Thank you for listening, I can go back to sleep now and put out your fire."

You might be wondering, though, why do some bacteria or viruses proliferate and cause infections, and others do not? Or…why can micro-organisms be part of our normal flora and yet become pathogens?

Our experience working with clients has taught us that there is always a change in the energetics of the Immune System that proceeds the development of an auto-immune condition, allergy, or chronic infection.

The change in energy changes the relationship between the micro-organism and the body.

Our Immune System is supposed to draw a proverbial line in the sand and say, "You (micro-organisms) stay on that side of the line, and we'll stay on this side, and everyone will remain happy (and healthy)."

With an energetic change, the conversation changes to, "Y'all come on in! Let's party! We'll go create some chaos together and build some fires!"

The Immune System develops an exaggerated response. It is now contributing to the damage of the body as much as or more than the micro-organisms.

And this is also true for allergic responses to the proteins found in nature. For example, we have found allergies develop in our clients to things that were in their environment at the time an emotional trauma was imprinted on their body.

They have usually been through many different types of therapies to remove or desensitize themselves to the allergens, without much improvement.

We have found that after using Sonic Alignment to release the energetic imbalance (caused by the emotional trauma) that started the reaction, their Immune System will respond to techniques such as Immunotherapy more readily.

Immune suppression (meaning the loss of various Immune System functionality) is usually no longer necessary.

Autoimmunity

In the late 1990's, I had the privilege of spending time, at an allergy conference, with Dr. Leonard McEwen, a brilliant immunologist from Great Britain. He forever changed my perspective on what auto-immunity is.

Dr. McEwen had been doing work with bacterial antigens and found that a number of autoimmune conditions were triggered by these microbial proteins. Dr. William "Butch" Shrader and other physicians in the American Academy of Environmental Medicine have continued his work in the US. It is known as low dose antigen therapy or LDA.

Rheumatoid diseases, such as rheumatic heart disease, have long been known to be associated with streptococcus infections. Even after the acute infection has cleared, the immune system starts attacking another area of the body: a joint, the skin, kidney, or heart valves, for example.

But why do these reactions occur in some people and not others?

I was taught in medical school that certain inherited patterns of protein expression are associated with an increased risk of rheumatic disease (major histocompatability antigens or MHA). I often wondered why these MHA groups have higher incidences in certain areas of the world and in certain family lines.

Could there be an environmental or other shared experience factor?

As Elena and I have worked together on clients with autoimmunity, we have found a change in the relationship between our client's immune system and one of the "passenger" microbes underlying the development of their autoimmune disease. This usually occurred at an emotionally charged time of their life. Their immune system has changed from its guardian "watch dog" role with the microbes, to a "Hey, let's go create some chaos and build a fire somewhere" relationship.

Conventional therapies focus on attacking the microbes with prescription or natural antimicrobials and suppression of the immune system. We have found, however, that removal of the energetic memory of the traumatic event precipitating the symptom flare-up, followed by a restoration of normal immune function, using Dr. McEwen's methods, to be effective in a wide variety of inflammatory conditions. Bacteria, fungi and viruses can act as triggers. When we have identified the correct triggers, symptoms start to improve within days.

Chronic Pain

Pain is a component of many of the disease processes that our clients present to us. With all the advancements in our knowledge of how the human body works, we still know very little about the mechanisms of pain and have no way to quantify or measure it other than with analog scales (For example, clients are asked, "On a scale of 1 to 10, how is your pain?"). However, one person's 7 is another person's 5. A stimulus that is painful to someone, may tickle another. You see the problem?

Instead of viewing pain as a neurochemical reaction of the body to a noxious stimulus, we see it as an indicator of disruption in energy flow or an alarm from the fight/flight/withdrawal system of the body. Frequently, it's both.

We identify the causes of the loss of energy flow in the body using Sonic Alignment and then make recommendations to restore function. This usually includes release of emotional energies, correction of dental issues, neutralization of scar tissues and restoring a balanced relationship with our client's microbes.

Frequently, we find an imbalance in the Sympathetic (fight or flight) and Parasympathetic (rest, digest, restore) nervous systems which regulate our body's function moment-to-moment. Areas of the body can get "stuck" in fight or flight resulting in reduced blood flow, muscle tension and loss of function. Pain is a side effect of this reaction. We use techniques to reset the balance between these two systems, reducing the fight/flight response and increasing the body's ability to rest and restore function.

When we use this combined approach with clients with chronic pain, our results have produced significant reductions in pain, frequently before the session has finished.

Chronic Infection

For more than 30 years, I have been waging war with microbes as an Otolaryngologist (Ear, Nose and Throat Specialist). I attended courses on infectious disease, learned about all the different antibiotics, how they work and how to combine them to get even better results.

However, despite all my best efforts, when it came to chronic infections, the bugs kept winning. They would either change and become resistant to the drugs I had chosen, or shortly after the drugs were stopped, when everything looked clear, a completely different organism would show up.

I would try surgery to open pathways for the body to drain or clear the infections. Some clients showed improvement. A few got worse.

As I began understanding more about Energy Medicine, I realized that the microbes were there because of a low energy condition. They were doing what they normally do in nature, cleaning up the trash. I called a truce to the war I was waging with them.

I also started to recognize that most of the damage and symptoms associated with chronic infection were not caused by the microbes. They were caused by the immune system's reaction to the microbes.

Many of these organisms, like staph and strep, are considered normal flora, in other words, bugs that belong on our spaceship human. So, what causes our immune system to go nuts when it encounters these bacteria instead of saying, "Have a nice day, but stay in your territory"?

Please don't misunderstand my intent. People with no immune system can succumb to overgrowth of multiple organisms, leading to their demise. The bacteria can do damage. I am referring more to an over-exaggerated response by the immune system. One that has "jumped the rails," so to speak.

Elena and I have worked with many clients who have been battling chronic infections for years with conventional and alternative health care. We have found that progress is not made until you stop battling the microbes, and, instead, restore harmony with the immune system. We have seen chronic symptoms resolve very rapidly and hope for the future return.

Headaches

When I was practicing Ear, Nose and Throat medicine, I used to have a programmable sign in front of my office. One of the things I advertised was the ability to relieve a headache in under a minute. It caused the local neurologists – the headache specialists – to call me a quack!

For more than 15 years, I have been successful at least 90% of the time lessening headache severity and, many times, completely alleviating the discomfort. It worked for migraine, cluster, and non-specific headaches, particularly in the front of the head.

A few years ago, I decided to get brave and try this in front of an audience. To begin my talk at a medical conference in Dallas, I invited anyone in the audience with a headache to come up. Since headaches are fairly common, I soon had three people volunteer. Most of them had already taken something earlier that day for their pain. All three were women: a teenager, a middle aged-woman and a professor in her forties from Harvard. I had each one grade the severity of their headache on a 1 to 10 scale with 5 being "Where's the pill bottle?" and 10 being "The worst headache I've ever had or could imagine." Their scores were between 5 and 8.

I had someone in the audience start a timer.

I used a dilute solution of a common, naturally occurring biochemical messenger and administered 1/10th of a cc (about 3 drops) under each person's tongue. I had them count to 10 and then swallow. I then had them grade the severity of their headache again. Two of them no longer had any headache. The third was given another 1/10th cc of a slightly different dilution of the same solution. After 10 more seconds, I asked her to grade her headache. It was gone. Three headaches gone, in less than a minute. I had everyone's attention for the rest of my talk.

So, what was in the solution I used?

A super strong pain killer?

A new wonder drug I made in my home chemistry lab?

Nope. It was a very dilute solution of something already in each of our bodies. Something that actually belonged there, but was "out of control". What I gave them acted like "noise cancellation," and their pain went away.

Back Pain

Many of our clients suffer from back pain. They may have had an injury from a motor vehicle accident, from lifting something too heavy, or perhaps from just turning the wrong way. Frequently, they have had other treatments for their back pain before they meet us. These include chiropractic therapies, acupuncture, massage, and even back surgery. These treatments may have provided temporary improvements, but no permanent resolution.

When we check the area of their back pain, we always find changes in the energy of that area which occurred long before any injury or symptoms of pain developed. Abnormal energy patterns can even be present at conception, indicating a contribution from the ancestors of the client. They can change in utero due to an emotional event the mother had during her pregnancy that transferred to the developing fetus. Or they can be acquired from adverse events during the client's lifetime.

Regardless of when the energy changes occur, the bladder meridians are usually involved with back pain.

The bladder acupuncture meridian is the longest energy meridian of the body. It begins between the eyes, traveling up between the eyebrows, over the top of the head, down the back of the neck, down the back, on either side of the spine, to the sacrum. It then jumps back up to the shoulders and comes down the back a second time, more laterally, just inside the shoulder blades, down to the buttocks, down the back of the legs to the outside of the foot, ending on the little toes.

Symbolically, the bladder meridian energy has to do with how we feel about our territory, our boundaries, our comfort zone, our space. Animals, for example, use their urine to mark their space or territory. We don't pee around the edges of our property, but we get "pissed off" when people don't respect or violate our boundaries.

We have found that our clients with back issues are in Fight-Flight-Freeze mode most of the time (also known as the Sympathetic portion of the Autonomic Nervous System) This is also the function of the bladder meridian. Fear of danger, injury, or destruction is at the root of this response. It allows us to survive, in the same way it allowed our ancestors to survive and pass on their responses to us through their DNA energy.

When you scare a cat, where does the hair stand up?

On its back, along the spine, over the bladder meridian.

When a dog gets angry, where does its hair stand up?

On its neck, over the bladder meridian.

If you sufficiently scare a child, or even an adult, what do they lose control of?

Their bladder.

You get the picture?

Disruption in the flow of energy in the bladder meridian can result in changes in muscle tension, bony alignment of the vertebrae, and the shortening or tightening of the fascial tissues, which together, change the function and mobility of the spine.

Pain is a symptom of this loss of energy flow and function.

By making our clients aware of the circumstances changing the energy flow of their backs, they are able to release old patterns and establish new ones, restoring energy flow to chronically deprived regions.

Their pain usually dissolves, and they experience improved mobility and function.

Part IV

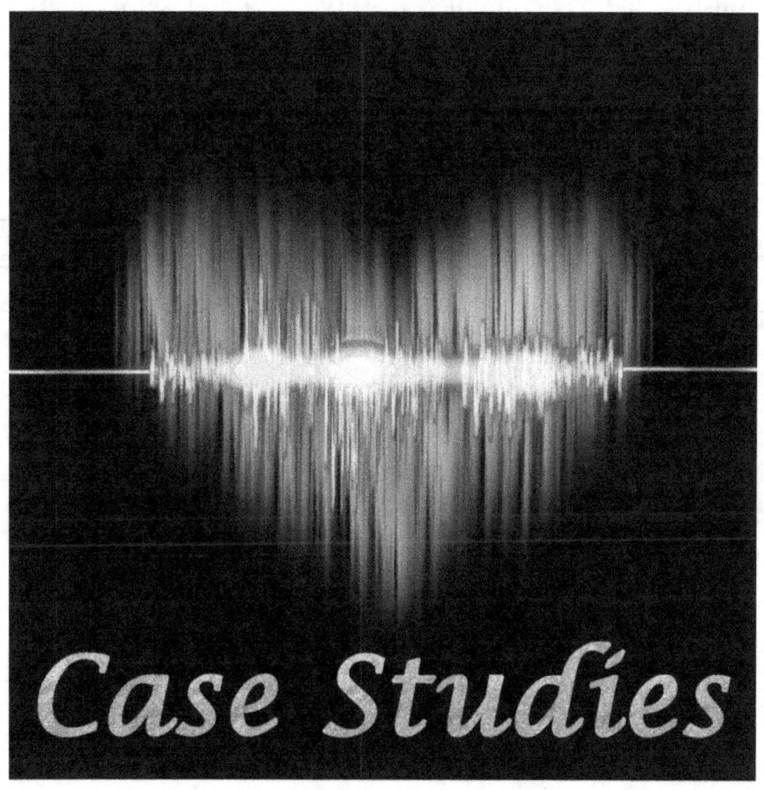

Chief Chuck and the Chuck Roast

On our first trip to visit Little Rock, Arkansas, our friend, Rev. Colleen, introduced us to her fiancé, Chief Chuck.

Colleen had sought us out after we had helped some of her friends and clients in Memphis, Tennessee. Since leaving her ministry, she has continued to serve as a counselor, helping clear emotional traumas and their psychological impact. Very open to the use of alternative methods and energy, she was impressed with the results we had helped her clients achieve with our Sonic Alignment methods.

Chuck is a retired Air Force Chief, the highest non-commissioned rank. Most of his friends call him "Chief". He even has an Indian Chief head on the front license plate of his car.

After leaving the Air Force, he worked with American Airlines for many years. He described his life as a baggage handler, loading heavy luggage into the bellies of jets. It had taken its toll on him physically. He had had two surgeries on his right shoulder and one on his left. Despite the two right shoulder surgeries, he still had pain and limitation of motion. He also had chronic pain in his right knee.

Chuck, at first, seemed quite skeptical about our techniques and abilities. He had not had the exposure to alternative healing methods that Colleen had. Because of Colleen's recommendation, though, he had agreed to try out a session with us.

Our evaluation found very heavy energy in his right shoulder, right knee and the right side of his mouth.

Examining his teeth one by one, we localized the problem to tooth #3 (the first molar on his upper right side).

The sound frequency we experienced was similar for all three areas, especially the tooth and the right shoulder. We recognized the sound of streptococcus.

Streptococcus, besides causing acute infections, can trigger auto-immune, rheumatoid reactions in the body. We have found it contributing to chronic inflammation of joints in many of our clients. Streptococcus is plentiful in the mouth and usually associated with dental problems.

We had Chuck open his mouth, and we saw that there was a filling in tooth #3, but no other obvious abnormality. He told us he had no symptoms in the tooth and was very skeptical that we had found a problem.

"I don't have any pain in that tooth and never have," he said, "but I'll tell you what, we'll find out just how good you are. I have a dentist's appointment tomorrow."

A slight look of fear came over Elena's face.

The next day we were at Colleen's home working with some of her other friends when Chuck returned from the dentist. He immediately summoned us into the kitchen.

"Well, I'll be darned", he said. "You were right! I didn't say anything to my dentist about what you said. She immediately noticed a problem with tooth #3. When she first looked, she said there was a small fracture at the gum line. She then took x-rays and found the tooth completely broken in half, deeper down, with infection in the bone around the tooth. She told me it would have to come out!"

He was so excited we had found a problem that could explain many of the issues he had with his health. He invited us to dinner at his home that night to say thank you. He had prepared a wonderful meal in his slow cooker: carrots, potatoes, onions, and of course, Chuck roast.

It was delicious.

Sonic Alignment for Professional Athletes

Having played sports professionally myself, I've always wondered if there might be an energetic reason or an inherited weakness that plays a contributing factor in an athlete sustaining an injury. Recently, after talking to a professional beach volleyball player, I realized that this can be true.

She had been struggling with an injury to one of her hamstrings. I asked her a couple of questions and determined there was indeed an emotional trauma related to lack of trust and feelings of not being in control. (These are emotions which affect the function of the bladder meridian, the power supply to the hamstrings.) She was amazed by the insights I was able to give to her. She had no idea her personal life was having such an effect on her physical performance.

In order to restore optimal function of the muscle, we believe that both the energetic and emotional components need to be addressed. Ultimately, we believe it is possible to improve strength and function to a higher degree than even before an injury. This is because there is usually an energetic blockage in the area long before the injury which has predisposed that area of the body to injury.

I was able to make recommendations to the beach volleyball player, which included changes in her training techniques. To increase her levels of trust and confidence, I recommended doing lunges in reverse through an obstacle course, while guided by the voice of her coach behind her. She would have to practice trust, while using those muscles.

We feel that injuries are not accidental. They are a weakness that has been waiting to fail.

A message from your body.

In my 30's, I lost my mother due to a stroke. I continued to carry grief for many years in my lung meridian (before I learned the principles that we're sharing with you). The lung meridian crosses the shoulder.

I have played professional and high-level amateur volleyball for over 30 years. And I've never had a shoulder injury.

But that doesn't make sense, does it?

Well…actually, it does make sense…

If I had been left-handed, the side where I carried my grief, then I am sure I would have been more likely to have an injury there.

Sonic Alignment can help identify why and where an area of the body became weak in the first place. It also empowers the athlete with the information he or she needs to address the affected area at both an energetic and physical level.

Most importantly, it helps the athlete develop the mental strength needed to build focus, self-esteem and self-trust, which can highly enhance performance.

Furry Friends

We've had several clients ask if we could help them with health or behavioral issues with their house pets. Because the same universal principles apply to the energy of animals, we have been successful in identifying the root cause of their pets' symptoms and have been able to provide guidance towards resolution.

Many pets are now rescued and have been exposed to very traumatic circumstances in their early life. Just like humans, these traumatic imprints affect the way they react to and interact with the world around them.

Using Sonic Alignment, we can pinpoint when in their lives the trauma occurred and the area of their body being affected. We can then help realign their energetic imprint.

The following experience will illustrate these principles:

One of our clients, Chelsea, in Southern Florida, asked us to evaluate her cat, Charlie. He had been having recurrent problems with his bladder and a lot of anxiety for the previous two weeks. The traditional remedies from their veterinarian weren't working, and they were getting concerned.

The cat was a stray who followed them home while they were out walking one day. They decided to call him Charlie. He had been a member of their family for more than six years.

He had recurrent problems with his urinary system, particularly his bladder. He would make frequent, unproductive trips to the litter box. In 2014, he had to have his bladder flushed. The veterinarian said he had never seen so much "grit" come out of one cat. He came home from the vet with a respiratory infection.

When his urinary symptoms flared, he'd also have behavioral changes in which he was at first lethargic, then start racing around and become skittish, not wanting to be touched.

A couple of years back, he'd had a similar flare up.

What we found when we evaluated him was a lot of fear in his lungs and the bladder meridian. We identified the timeline of the development of his current symptoms, down to the day, and the prior occurrence as well. We then checked to see when the first pattern had appeared. It was at conception, which meant he had an inherited pattern from one of his parents. We found the same frequency in his mother, close to her birth in 2004.

In Chinese Medicine, fear is associated with the bladder meridian. The meridian begins at the inside corners of the eyes, runs up the forehead, over the top, and down the back, along the spine. When you scare a cat, that's where the hair stands up. If you frighten a human, they will lose control of their bladder.

While we were working on Charlie, he hid in the curtains, trying to wrap himself up in them. When we finished, he jumped up on the bed and started purring.

Elena had a strong feeling it was something in the environment that was responsible for all these reactions.

Can you guess what might scare a cat in Southern Florida?

All the time points were when hurricanes were threatening Florida. The most recent flare up began when Hurricane

Dorian was approaching Miami. We looked up the name of the hurricane in 2004, the one that started the pattern in Charlie's mother, and to our amazement it was – Charlie!

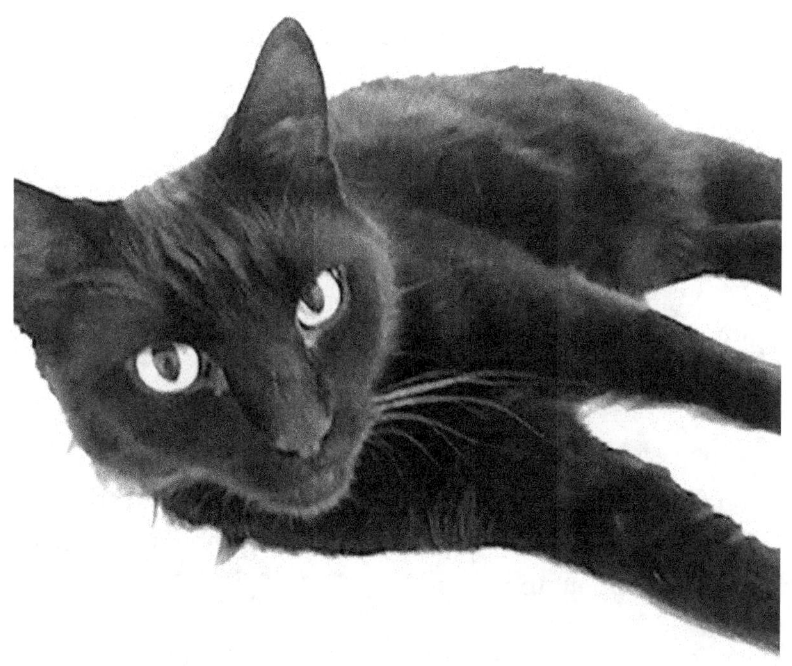

Charlie

(Note: Look at the inside corners of Charlie's eyes, where the bladder meridian starts. See the yellow collections there?!)

Charlie is a 7-year-old male cat with a history of urinary issues. We keep a close eye on his behavior and litter box habits. He was alternating between lethargy and "the zoomies", acting skittish, avoiding touch, and visiting the litter box frequently.

Two vet visits in two months resulted in two rounds of prescription medication. Charlie hated the meds. He hid from us at dosage time and squished his ears to avoid the transdermal cream. It was hard to tell if the meds even relieved his symptoms.

Dr. Hyde and Elena to the rescue! We set up a tele-session on September 15, 2019. Charlie hung out in the room before the session officially began— almost like he knew something good was about to happen.

None of Charlie's history was shared before the session. We simply sent a photo of him. Dr. Hyde and Elena walked us through significant events in Charlie's life— identifying his emotions and affected organs. Several remedies were suggested. (He has accepted half of them, which is pretty good for a cat.)

Over the six weeks since the session, Charlie is more social and affectionate. His playfulness returned — even playing fetch with his toy mouse. He acts less skittish when there is a loud noise. And litter box frequency is way down. (These observations were also made by someone who does not know about the tele-session. She spends a lot of time with Charlie and keeps tabs on his behavior for us.)

We are delighted Charlie is healthy again! Much gratitude for Dr. Hyde and Elena for sharing their very special healing skills with us.

Horse Health

Two of our dear friends have a small farm in Texas where they take-in working horses, such as polo ponies and rodeo horses, who have become lame. They give them tender loving care during the final years of their life. We love going to their farm to enjoy the quiet solitude and loving spirit that abounds there.

During one of our first visits to their farm, they asked if we could evaluate their horses. One of them, Elizabeth, was very nervous and would not allow most humans to get close to her.

We had not tried our techniques on horses yet, but were curious what we could identify and do to possibly help. So, tuning forks in hand, we headed out to the field.

As we approached Elizabeth, she would walk away from us, always keeping a distance of twenty feet or more between us. She was visibly nervous and had a scared look in her eyes.

After several attempts to approach her, talking in low, non-threatening tones, we decided we had to find another way to get close to her. So, we closed our eyes and imagined we were standing next to her. There...we were able to connect with her energy.

Elena and I scanned her body. Elena found a lot of blocked energy around her face and neck, and she heard the sound of pain. It started early in her life, around the time when training would normally begin. She had been a polo pony. We learned later from her owners that some trainers will strike a horse in the face and neck during training.

We worked to realign the energy in the area and lift the fearful imprint from her. After working for several minutes, we opened our eyes. She was standing much closer to us. We closed our eyes again and continued working this way, until we felt all the disturbances had been cleared. When we opened our eyes the final time, Elizabeth was standing next to us, less than an arm's length away.

For the rest of our visit at the farm, Elizabeth would be waiting for us whenever we went outside and would follow us as we went around the property. Elena once got in the golf cart and went exploring around the property, and Elizabeth followed her everywhere she went. As Elena went through some brush around a corner, though, Elizabeth stopped following her. Elena thought that was strange. She continued around the corner to find it came to a dead end at the edge of the property. Elena turned the cart around and as she came back out of the brush, there was Elizabeth waiting, with a look on her face as if she were saying, "I knew you would be back."

Elizabeth remained much calmer and no longer showed her distrust of humans. We visited the farm several more times over the next year, and she came right up to us each time, allowing us to pet her and feed her carrots.

We also worked on some of their other horses, including Einstein and Duke. Duke had been a rodeo cutting horse. He had become lame in his right hind leg. As we worked on him, we found out there was an energy block in the upper leg due to a scar. The scar was caused by a brand with a large block "G". Duke and the other horses had other brands on them, but they didn't seem to affect the energy like this one.

We tracked the timeline of the change to when the brand was placed and found the same negative energy in the person who had branded Duke. His energy had transferred to the horse and into the wound. We have found similar transferred energies in some of the surgical scars of our human clients.

With the supervision of a veterinarian, we used a German technique known as Neural Therapy to clear the energy from the scar. As soon as we finished, Duke started putting more weight on his right rear hoof.

We noticed on our last visit to their farm that the large block "G" is no longer visible, at all!

As for Einstein…

He has a very unusual coat for a horse. It's actually curly, kind of like a poodle. I joked that he was a cross between a horse and poodle. Elena later "heard" that he didn't like my comment.

When we worked on Einstein, we found that his main problem was that he didn't like the skin he was in. (We've had human clients who manifested different skin disorders varying from psoriasis to skin cancer who had similar emotions to Einstein.)

As a result of his attitude, Einstein constantly tries to draw attention to himself. When we feed the horses, he pushes in front of the others, and if he feels we are not giving him enough attention, he acts out.

We try to give him unconditional love and enjoy his quirky behavior. As a result, he has been much more friendly with us.

When we were trying to leave the farm, Einstein and Duke decided they didn't want us to go. Einstein stood in front of our car. Elena rolled down her window to try to persuade

Einstein to move. When she did so, Duke tried to put his head through her window. We had to go get some carrots to get them to move. *Maybe they were training us?*

Acknowledgement

Whenever you try something new, it takes a lot of courage.

That courage has to come from somewhere. It has to be nurtured.

This is our first experience writing a book. It is very frightening. You feel very vulnerable.

We feel strongly writing is something we need to do. The understanding we are receiving won't continue unless we are willing to share it.

You have to give in order to receive.

Thank God for coaches! They help you avoid making messy mistakes and help you find the courage to accomplish what you had only a glimmer of hope of achieving.

Our writing coach is an amazing woman! She is an incredible human being!

Her unflappable optimism and encouragement kept us going through our times of self-doubt and self-criticism. She helped us find our voice and gain confidence in our ability to speak through the written word.

We encourage anyone who feels they have a book inside them to connect with her.

Thank you, D. D. Scott, and the team at letloveglow.com.

Note from The Authors

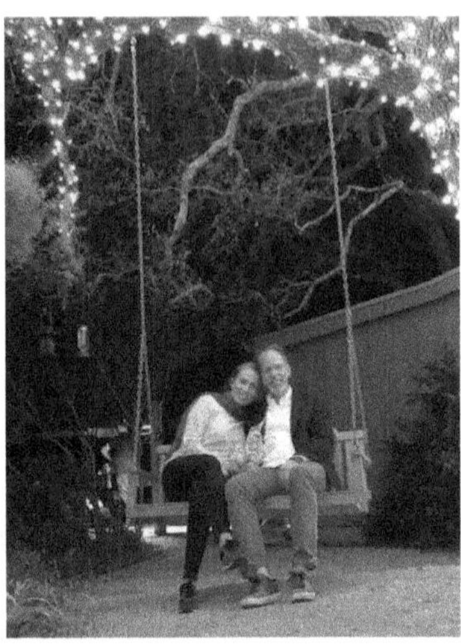

Thank you for your interest in our work. We love what we do.

We are overwhelmed by the love and acceptance we receive from our clients every day. It takes a lot of courage and trust to become vulnerable to who you really are. It's hard to love your weaknesses and imperfections so they can become your strengths.

Our clients are great examples to us.

We are looking at the world through child-like eyes, seeing things for the first time that have been there all along.

We are listening and recognizing the song of frequencies that are inherent in everything and everyone.

We will continue to write and share the knowledge we receive as we work with our clients.

It is not our knowledge. It is the intelligent pattern of life.

Future books in this series will explain our emotional relationships with additional minerals, vitamins, neurotransmitters, hormones, microbes, and toxins. This is just a start!

We have found some unique ways to interface with life. Our goal is to teach others so they can bring their unique qualities to further this work with us.

If this resonates with you, please join us on this incredible journey of discovery.

If this is not your journey, but you know someone who is on this path, please share this book with them.

You can reach us by email at happytohelp@vita.science. We would love to hear from you and what you liked and didn't like about our book.

We want to learn from every experience. Making mistakes is the human experience.

Please leave us a review on the site or store where you found our book. Your vote of confidence will give others who need our message courage and hope.

We will be posting health tours, educational events, and upcoming publications on our websites and social media.

Connect with us on the following:

Dr. Greg
* https://www.facebook.com/drgreghyde
* https://www.instagram.com/drghyde/

Elena
* https://www.facebook.com/profile.php?id=100014051793484
* https://www.instagram.com/elenamerani/

Dr. Greg and Elena
* https://vita.science
* https://sonicalignment.com

* facebook.com/theVitaInstitute

Many blessings,

Dr. Greg & Elena

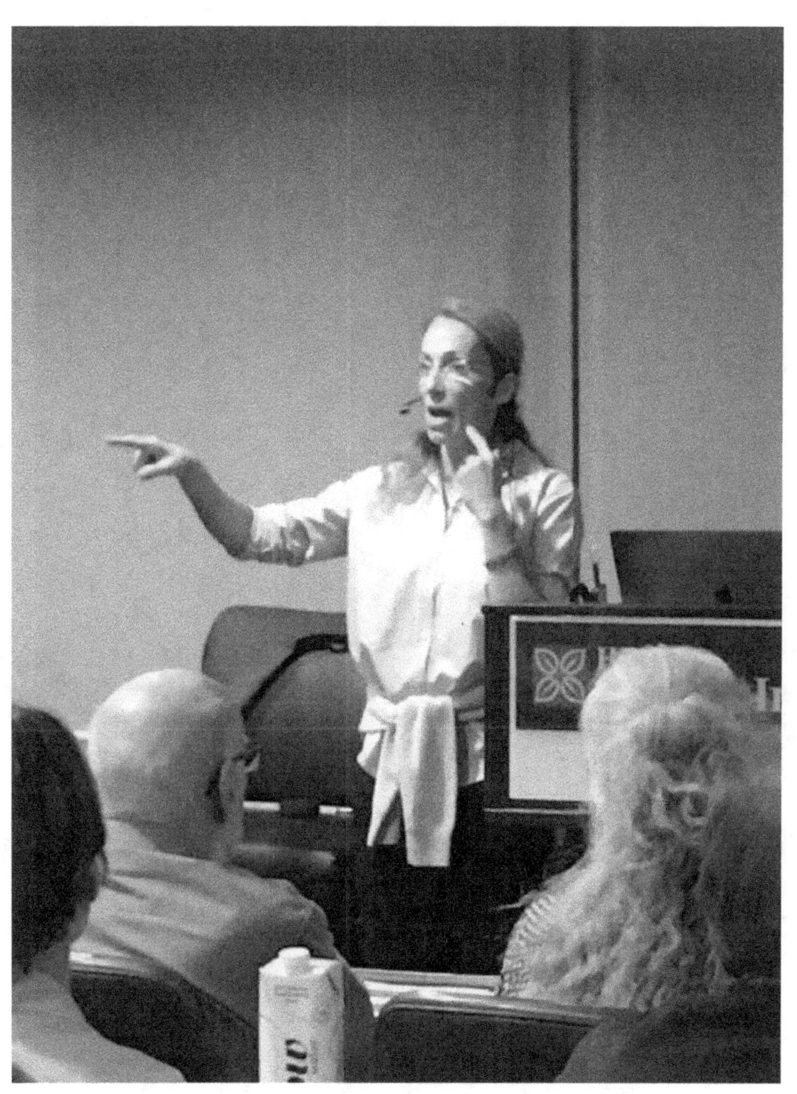

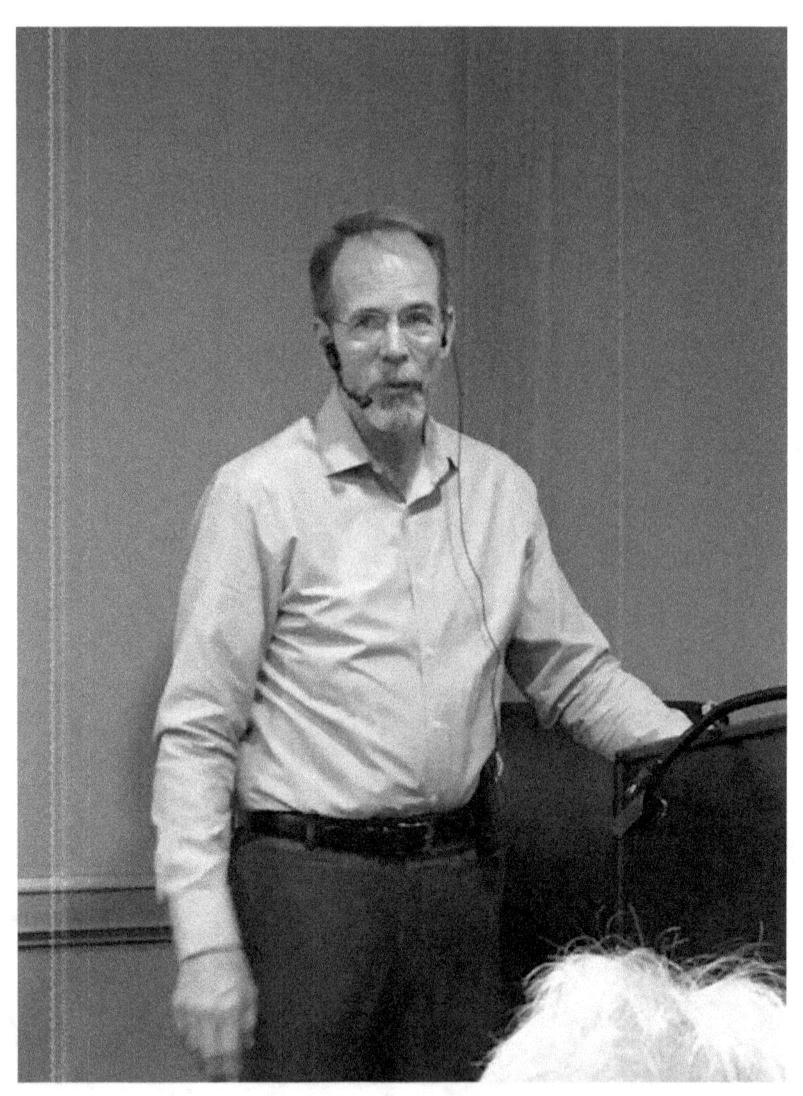

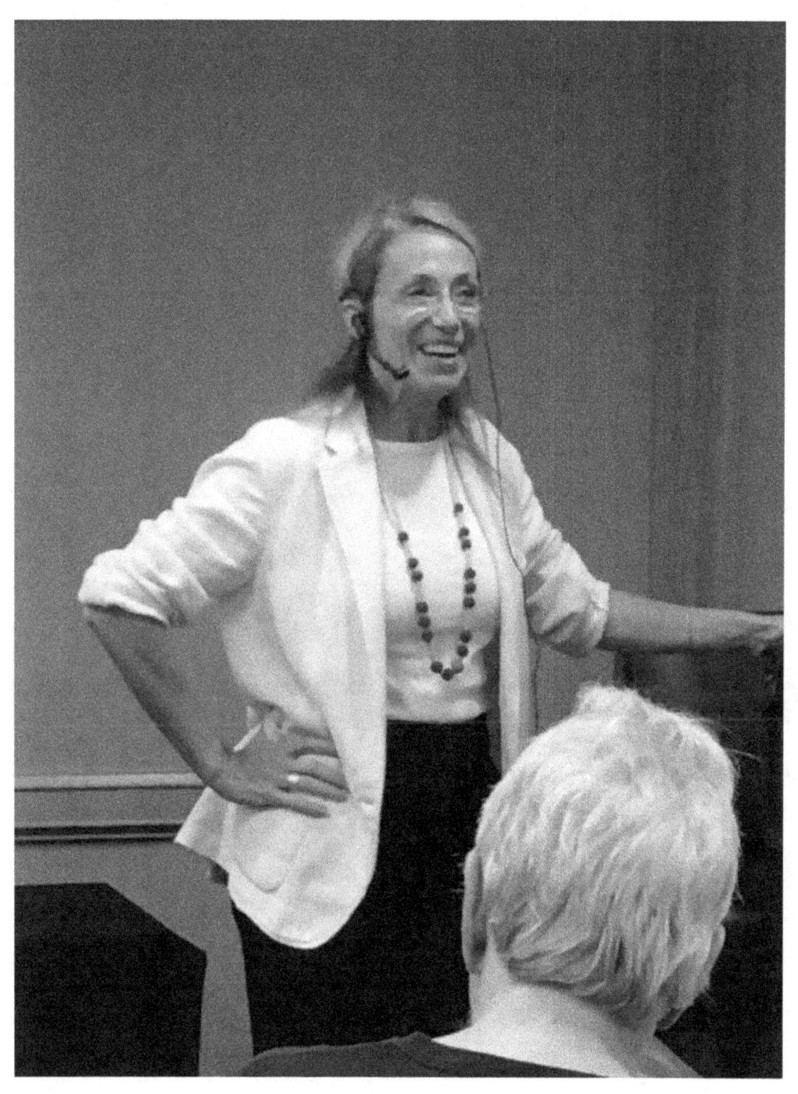

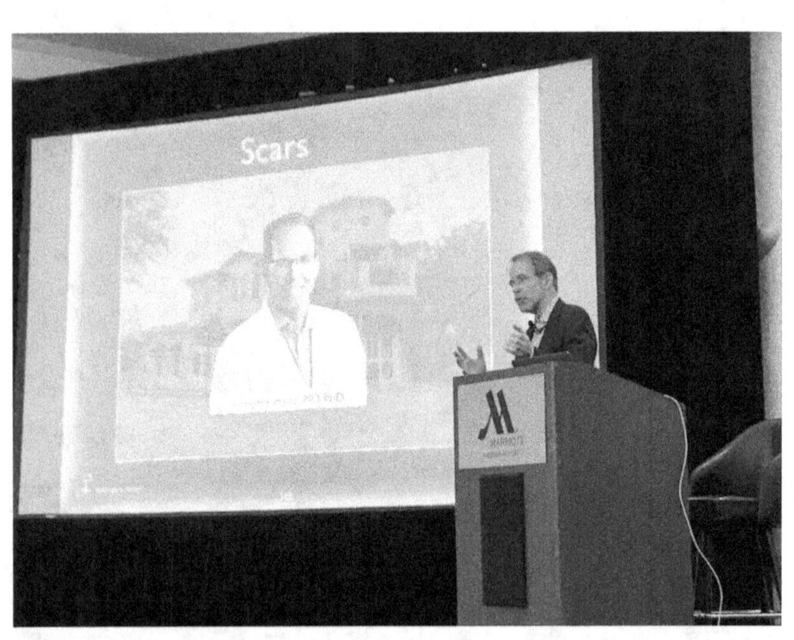

Scars

About The Authors

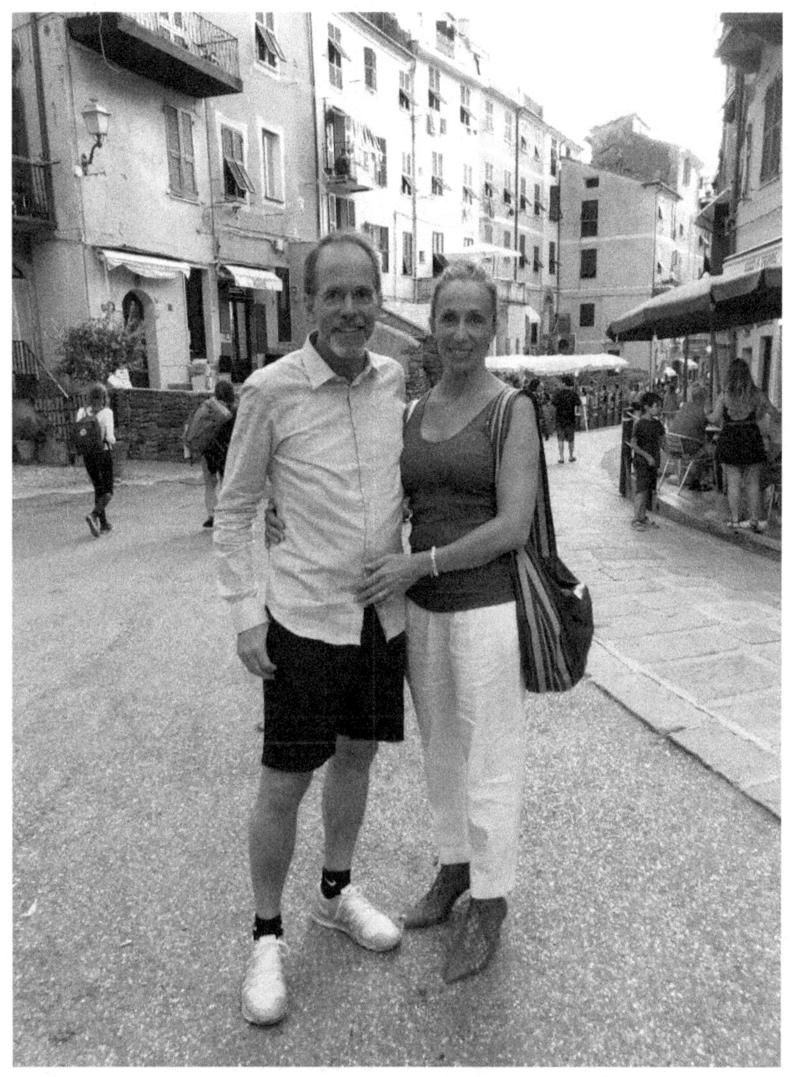

**Gregory Hyde, M.D., PhD
and Elena Merani, ND, CNHP**

Greg and Elena bring together their knowledge to empower people in their journey of self-healing. Their gentle dance guides those who are ready, towards the discovery of their truth.

Greg and Elena are not healers. They help people open the doors to opportunities which allow the healing process to manifest.

Elena studied science and languages in Italy. She became a Naturopath in 2010, and now practices Sonic Alignment with her husband, as well as Biofield Tuning and other emotional release modalities. Elena loves to observe the beauty and potential in people. She enjoys singing and dancing with her husband and creating foods for your emotions. It's all about cooking, dancing and great shoes…you can't take the Italian out of her!

Greg is an MD with a PhD in Neuroscience from the University of Washington in Seattle. He has strong backgrounds in Chemistry, Allergy/Immunology, Endocrinology, Environmental, Regenerative, and Sleep Medicine. He has over 25 years of experience in Integrative and Alternative healing practices.

He loves to cook healthy meals, sing, and dance with his wife, Elena. His personal passion is developing home and work environments which inherently increase life force and encourage self-healing through the use of correct building materials, lighting, color, and sacred geometry.

Since 2017, they have been developing a technique they call Sonic Alignment. It uses coherent sound to identify imbalances in the body. During the development of this technique, Elena recognized that the sound of many emotions matches the sound of an element in The Periodic Table. Emotional frequencies have corresponding mineral frequencies.

There is a Periodic Table of Emotions.

Dr. Greg and Elena have found that mineral imbalances are related to emotional imbalances. Together, they observe how life experiences, genetic patterns, thoughts and emotions affect the subtle balance of the elements that make up our bodies and the world around us.

Sharing this knowledge with clients has allowed the recipients to re-establish the correct relationship with their minerals and vital elements and regain their function.

Life is relationships.

Books by the Authors

<u>HEALING WITH SOUND
AND THE PERIODIC TABLE OF EMOTIONS:</u>

Healing with Sound and The Periodic Table of Emotions (Volume I)

Our Quantum Relationship with Water: Why Sonic Alignment Works (Volume II) – *Coming Soon!*